THEORETICAL
FOUNDATIONS
OF
NURSING

GERTRUDE TORRES

THEORETICAL FOUNDATIONS OF NURSING

APPLETON-CENTURY-CROFTS/Norwalk, Connecticut

ISBN: 0-8385-8945-6

Copyright © 1986 by Appleton-Century-Crofts
A Publishing Division of Prentice-Hall, Inc.

86 87 88 89 90 91/10 9 8 7 6 5 4 3 2 1

Prentice-Hall International (UK) Limited, *London*
Prentice-Hall of Australia Pty. Limited, *Sydney*
Prentice-Hall Canada Inc., *Toronto*
Prentice-Hall Hispanoamericana, S.A., *Mexico*
Prentice-Hall of India Private Limited, *New Delhi*
Prentice-Hall of Japan, Inc., *Tokyo*
Prentice-Hall of Southeast Asia Pte. Ltd., *Singapore*
Editora Prentice-Hall do Brasil, Ltda., *Rio de Janeiro*
Whitehall Books Limited, *Wellington, New Zealand*

Library of Congress Cataloging-in-Publication Data

Torres, Gertrude.
    Theoretical foundations of nursing.

    Bibliography; p.
    Includes index.
    1. Nursing—Philosophy. I. Title. [DNLM:
1. Models, Theoretical. 2. Philosophy, Nursing.
WY 86 T693t]
RT84.5.T67 1986   610.73'01   85-15037
ISBN 0-8385-8945-6

Editorial/production supervision: Fay Ahuja
Interior design: Eleanor Henshaw Hiatt
Cover design: Wanda Lubelska Design
Manufacturing buyer: John B. Hall

To Virginia Carley,
a Grey Nun of the Sacred Heart
—a friend—
an inspiration to all who know her

CONTENTS

PREFACE

The major purpose of this book is to give the reader an understanding of the development and status of nursing theories. Within the last ten years many texts have been written that have been oriented toward explaining and describing either a specific theory or multiple theories in nursing. For the most part, their approach has been to view each theory separately. This text differs in that four major themes by which to classify nursing theories are identified—environment, need, systems, and interaction. The theme approach offers the reader the opportunity to compare, contrast, integrate, and analyze each of the theories.

The text has three areas of focus. Chapters 1 through 6 provide the foundation on which each of the theories will be discussed. Chapter 1 introduces the reader to the historical development of seventeen nursing theories and identifies the major themes and the emphasis of each theory.

Chapter 2 focuses on the understanding of theory, the development of theory, and methods of evaluating theories. Understanding of this chapter is central to the text, because the terminology defined is used throughout the book. Chapter 3 provides a basic understanding of the nursing process so that the use of each theory within a clinical situation can be discussed later in the text. These chapters do not provide an in-depth approach to theory or the nursing process, since other texts can be used that are separately oriented toward those areas.

Chapters 4 through 7 focus on the major theories. Except for the environment theme (Chapter 4) all others chapters first present the scientific or foundational writings that have influenced the development of the theories that follow; this facilitates understanding and comparison. Each theory is presented as follows: an overview of the major concepts is provided, models are developed, the use of the theory in relation to the nursing process is described, and the theory is evaluated. At the end of each chapter, there is a discussion of the integration of the theories.

The placement of any specific theory within a theme is often obvious—Henderson's theory categorized as a need theory, for example. On the other hand, identifying a theorist such as Hall within the interaction theme emphasizes more than the interactive approach to nursing care. Thus, the specific placement of a particular theorist within a theme is somewhat arbitrary but serves the purpose of the text.

Chapter 8 reviews the major concepts identified within all seventeen theories and offers a model for review. Propositions that appear basic to all theories are identified.

Within the text the term *patient* or *client* is used depending mostly upon how the particular theorist approached the individual; the term *man* is used with the same rationale.

The author is most grateful to the theorists for their contributions to nursing, and to Helen Yura, Dorothy Ozemek, Suzanne Falco, and Janie Brown Nowak who were very helpful in their reviews of the text. The author also thanks Sr. Nancy Kaczmarek for her technical assistance and Maria Cotroneo for her support in getting the manuscript typed. Thanks also to Nancy Andreola for her careful and conscientious editing.

Acknowledgement must also go to Dr. Peggy L. Chinn, who encouraged me to write the text, and to my students at D'Youville College, who facilitated my thinking about nursing theory.

THEORETICAL
FOUNDATIONS
OF
NURSING

1

HISTORICAL PERSPECTIVES
IN THE DEVELOPMENT
OF NURSING THEORY

INTRODUCTION

The main purpose of knowing our past is to give us a clearer understanding of our present. History helps us understand our *patterns
of change* and the *evolution of ideas*. Knowledge does not exist
in a static form. We are constantly adding to what we know or believe to be true. Within a discipline there appear to be periods during
which a great deal of new knowledge is generated; at other times the
pace may seem quite slow. The perception of this pace is strongly
influenced by the degree and extent to which the members of the
discipline incorporate the new knowledge into their practice.

Over the last 120 years, nursing has developed a body of knowledge, the major purpose of which has been to explain the practice of
nursing as different and distinct from the practice of medicine. Nursing's major theme has consistently focused on *the understanding of
human beings within their environment in relation to their needs*.
This theme can be identified within all nursing theories. The terminology may differ at times, but the focus remains the same. This emphasis has functioned as a guide for the evolution of ideas in nursing.
From a historical point of view, we find common elements

within all the nursing theories based on certain assumptions, such as the following:

Human beings will benefit from nursing care.

Human beings have an inner capacity to improve their health state.

An increased understanding of human beings will facilitate and improve nursing care.

Nursing knowledge relates to the state of human health and disease.

Nursing practice is distinct from other health care professions.

Human beings interact with each other.

Human beings do not exist in isolation—they are influenced by individuals, families, and environment.

The health of human beings consists of more than their biological needs.

Improved health is a goal of society.

Health is a positive value.

These assumptions are supported by the biological, psychological, and social sciences. The greater the knowledge of such sciences, the more the nurse will be able to understand and accept the nature of the human being and the appropriate role of the professional nurse. For example, a sound background in psychological theory provides a basis for the understanding of the interaction among the patient, the nurse, the family, and other health care workers.

In studying nursing theories, it is essential to see how they are similar, how they differ, and how one theory clarifies a previous one. Nursing theories build on previous knowledge either from science or from other nursing theories. New knowledge is not created in a vacuum but instead frequently reflects the synthesis and integration of old ideas into a more creative combination of thought. Thus, in viewing each of the theories, from Nightingale's to Watson's, one needs to search for ideas from the past upon which each theory has been built, and for ideas that present a different way of viewing nursing care.

Although we have the writings of seventeen nursing theorists, all but one of them were published after 1952. There may be several possible explanations for this recency. Nursing has paid little or no attention to the writings of Nightingale throughout history in terms of directing its practice. It is only recently that students across the country have been exposed to her book, *Notes on Nursing*. Thus, since the first theoretical base did not gain much visibility, little motivation existed for teachers and theorists of nursing to develop and publish their theories. There probably have been nursing leaders who created sound ideas about the understanding of human needs and the function of the nurse but who produced little written work. Even today we need to encourage many theorists to publish.

Table 1-1 identifies the nurse-theorists in chronological order, their themes, and the title that reflects their major orientation.

Basically, four major themes have evolved in nursing over the years: environment, need, interaction, and systems. In some theories, the theme is rather obvious and clear-cut, such as Nightingale's focus on the environment, and Henderson's emphasis on needs. In others, there is a greater thrust in the direction of a particular theme, but with a sort of integration of several themes. Examples are Rogers, who stresses the environment but also uses the systems approach, and Hall, who is oriented not only toward meeting the comfort needs of patients but also toward the interaction theme. This categorization serves a useful purpose for understanding and integrating nursing theories. However, the theme should not be viewed as simply reflecting a single approach by the theorist within her theory, but rather it should be seen as a way of organizing the *major* emphasis within the theory for review.

In reviewing Table 1-1, it is apparent that the three themes that have received the most attention are *needs, systems,* and *interaction*. The emphasis on *needs* was particularly significant from the mid-1950s to the mid-1960s, while *systems* gained momentum in the late 1960s and continues to be the strongest of the themes. The *interactive* theme can be identified in each decade; the *environmental* theme is given limited attention.

Increasingly, a greater number of theorists published their ideas. During the 1950s, two theorists published; during the 1960s, six published; and during the 1970s, eight published. At this pace, the number during the 1980s could easily reach over a dozen. This is a positive trend, although many would claim it adds to the confusion. On the contrary; since one theorist tends to build on others, and since there is a common focus on the distinct practice of nursing, additional theories serve to better explain nursing knowledge. This becomes increasingly evident as one reviews the theories throughout this book. The *environmental* theme emphasizes environmental surroundings and how they affect human beings. Nightingale focused on such things as air, light, noise, and smell, while Rogers speaks to the

Table 1-1

Themes and the Historical Development
of Nursing Theory

Date	Theorist	Environment	Need	Systems	Interaction
1860	Nightingale "Environment and Nature"	X			
1952	Peplau "Interpersonal Relation"				X
1955	Henderson "Human Needs"		X		
1960	Abdellah "Typology of Nursing Problems"		X		
1961	Orlando "Meeting Expressed Needs"		X		
1962	Hall "Cure, Care, Core"				X
1964	Wiedenbach "Realists in Nursing"		X		
1966	Levine "Conservative Principles"				X
1968	Johnson "Behavioral Systems"			X	
1970	Rogers "Unitary Man and Environment"			X	
1971	Orem "Self-Care Deficits"		X		
1971	King "Goal Attainment"			X	
1971	Travelbee "Interpersonal and Stress"				X
1972	Neuman "Open Systems Model; Stress and Reaction"			X	
1976	Roy "Adaptation"			X	
1977	Kinlein "Self-Care Practices and Health"		X		
1979	Watson "Humanistic, Altruistic, Interpersonal Process"				X

closeness of man-environment exchanging matter and energy. Thus, Nightingale's basic interest is the immediate environment, while Rogers more strongly addresses the totality of the world around humans.

The *need* theme is one of the strongest within nursing. Theorists use different terminology to express this theme, but the meaning is the same. For example, *Abdellah* uses the word *problem* to mean *need*; *Hall* relates to providing comfort; and *Orem* speaks of individuals' need for self-care. The major idea expressed within this theme is that of the nurse identifying some need on the part of the client and either meeting that need or assisting the client to meet it. The *interaction* theme developed by *Peplau* and *Travelbee* focuses on the patient and the nurse and views their relationship as a way of meeting needs or dealing with stress. These theorists tend to focus more on psychological needs than on biological ones.

The *systems* theme, more recently emphasized, tends to be somewhat more complex, bringing into play multiple ideas and their relationships. *Johnson* recognizes many subsystems or ideas—such as ingestion, aggression/protection, and dependency—that have a strong relationship to her major orientation toward behavioral systems. *King,* with her focus on goal attainment, finds relationships between perceptions, judgments, and interaction.

Table 1-2 identifies the theorists' ideas about the major role and function of nursing. In order to more clearly understand the history of the development of nursing knowledge, it is important to gain an understanding of each theorist's ideas about nursing and their implications for practice. Professional nursing can be practiced only when it is based on theory.

Table 1-2

Major Nursing Theorists' Ideas
on Nursing (1860–1981)

Nursing Theorist	Date	Identified Nursing Role and Function
Nightingale	1860	Facilitate nature's reparative process by providing an *environment* that will require the least expense of vital power on the part of the patient.
Peplau	1952	Provide an *interpersonal process* focusing on a felt need of the individual which is a determining force for the individual and the nurse.
Henderson	1955	Assist patient in meeting those of fourteen basic *needs* that he lacks strength to meet independently.
Abdellah	1960	Identify the problems of the patient within a twenty-one nursing problem classification system and provide total patient care to meet *needs.*

Table 1-2 (*cont.*)

Nursing Theorist	Date	Identified Nursing Role and Function
Orlando	1961	Interact with the patient to meet the immediate *need* for help by identifying the behavior of the patient, the reaction of the nurse, and the nursing action to be taken.
Hall	1962	Provide care and comfort to the patient during the disease process through exploration of the individual's concerns and through the *interactive* process.
Wiedenbach	1964	Assist individuals to overcome *obstacles* that interfere with their ability to meet the demands/*needs* brought about by a condition, environment, situation, or time.
Levine	1966	Intervene through human *interactions* to support and promote adjustments through four conservation principles of nursing, recognizing that individuals are dependent on relationships with others.
Johnson	1968	Foster efficient and effective *behavioral functioning* in the patient to prevent illness and during an episode of illness.
Rogers	1970	Focus on humanistic approaches that describe *unitary man,* environment, and the nature and direction of human development.
Orem	1971	Focus on the individual's *need* for *self-care* action in order to sustain life and health.
King	1971	Set and achieve *goals* based on nurse-client perceptions to help individuals maintain health in order to function in their roles.
Travelbee	1971	Assist individuals, families, and the community to prevent and cope with the *stress* of illness and to find meaning in the experience through an *interpersonal* process.
Neuman	1972	Reduce *stress* and adverse conditions through purposeful intervention that could have an effect on the patient's optimal functioning and state of wellness.
Roy	1976	Utilize the nursing process to manipulate *stimuli* to promote *adaptation.*
Kinlein	1977	Identify *self-care* practices as related to the patient's state of health.
Watson	1979	The science of nursing involves an *interpersonal process* which involves a humanistic-altruistic value-oriented approach.

Each theorist's definition of nursing has some similarities to and differences from the thinking of previous theorists, which are especially apparent when the theme is identified. For example, if we look at the *need* theme, *Henderson* focused on fourteen needs of the patient, *Abdellah* on twenty-one nursing problems that must be identified in order to meet patient needs, and *Orlando* on the immediate needs without specifically identifying them. Their similarity is reflected in their focus on need, and their differences in their enumeration of different needs. Generally, a nurse using any of these three theorists in practice would offer the patient similar nursing care. For example, if a patient requires fluids after surgery, all three theoretical approaches would lead the nurse to find ways of providing for fluid needs.

When we compare the definitions of nursing of theorists who focus on different themes, the major approach to providing nursing care could differ substantially. For example, while *Neuman* (systems theme) would focus on the environmental stressors that caused the patient to become ill and on the prevention of further stressors, *Orem* (need theme) would view individuals from the perspective of meeting their own self-care needs. Thus, in the case of the patient who needs fluids, *Neuman's* approach would identify the stressors that created that particular need, and *Orem* would identify ways that patients could meet their own need for fluids. Admittedly, no matter which theory one used, including *Peplau's* (interaction theme), the patient would have fluids. It is the nurse's total approach to the patient in relation to fluid needs that differs. *Orem* would ensure that patients could if possible meet their own needs for fluid, and *Neuman* would identify the stressors that are created if fluid needs are not met. It will become increasingly evident to you that in dealing with very specific needs of human beings, the theorists' ideas are hard to separate and the care is similar. When assessing the total patient and evaluating as much data as possible about the patient's situation, the theorists' differences and the impact that their approaches have on nursing care become increasingly evident. As is the case with psychological or teaching theories, different nursing theories do influence the nurse's total approach to care.

THEORY AND PRACTICE

Nursing theory is basic to professional nursing practice. Each theory provides a different way of viewing a particular patient-nurse situation. Table 1-3 identifies the focus of each theory and its potential use in a clinical situation involving a patient who has entered an emergency room. Only the highlights of the theories are presented here; later in the book a more detailed presentation of each will be given.

Table 1-3

Nursing Theory and Practice

Clinical Situation

An elderly woman has just entered the emergency room complaining of the difficulty she is having moving her right leg and arm. She was found on the floor of a food store no longer able to walk and was brought into the hospital by ambulance. She is very anxious and repeatedly reminds the nurse that her dog is alone in her apartment. She wants to call her neighbor to check her dog, and to return home so that she can care for her dog.

*Focus of Theory**	*Emphasis of Nursing Theory*	*Clinical Approach*
Nightingale (*Notes on Nursing*)	The proper environment for the patient "uses fresh air, light, warmth, cleanliness, quiet, and the proper selection and administration of diet—all at the least expense of vital power to the patient" (p. 8). Nursing focuses on creating a positive environment through the manipulation of the patient's surroundings in order to enhance the reparative process.	The nurse reviews the emergency room environment and finds that it is clean, warm, and well lighted. She places the woman in the quietest area to discuss her home environment with her. The nurse, at the request of the woman, calls a neighbor who is a close friend to watch the dog for her. Thus, the woman can now utilize her energies to assist in her own care.
Peplau (*Interpersonal Relations in Nursing*)	"Nursing is a significant, therapeutic, interpersonal process. Nursing is an educative instrument, a maturing force that aims to promote forward movement of personality in the direction of creative, constructive, productive personal and community living" (p. 16). The relationship has four phases: orientation, identification, exploration, and resolution, and is initiated by the recognition of a felt need which is related to a health problem.	The nurse identifies the woman's need to care for her pet at home and her need to become mobile. The nurse, acting as a counselor, identifies who can meet her need, contacts the neighbor, and resolves that concern. Both the nurse and the woman continue the relationship in a creative way either until the woman is mobile, or until she has matured in such a way as to accept her limitation.

Henderson
(*Textbook of Principles and Practice of Nursing*, with Harmer)

"Nursing is primarily assisting the individual (sick or well) in the performance of those activities contributing to health or its recovery (or a peaceful death) that he would perform unaided if he had the necessary strength, will or knowledge" (p. 4). This can be done by identifying the needs of the patient in terms of fourteen components.

The nurse allows the woman to express her fears and opinions, and assists her in caring for the dog by contacting the neighbor. Her fourteen needs are carefully reviewed, including her ability to breathe normally, eat and drink, eliminate, move, rest, maintain her body temperature, clean herself, avoid danger, communicate her needs, and deal with her faith, work, recreational, and learning needs. The focus of the care will be to aid the woman to become independent, especially in the area of bodily movement.

Abdellah
(*Patient-Centered Approaches to Nursing*)

Patient needs can be classified into four categories: sustenal care related to survival needs; remedial care directed toward restoring the patient's self-help ability by reducing or correcting the impaired state; restorative care helping the patient to live with impairment; and preventive care making the patients better able to help themselves (p. 51 and 52). These needs are reviewed from the framework of twenty-one nursing problems relating to the biological, psychological, and social needs of the patient.

After the nurse calls the neighbor, she will identify, under sustenal care, whether her needs for physical comfort, rest and activity, safety, oxygen, nutrition, fluids, and excretion are being met. She will focus on preventing complications from the patient's immobility and helping her live with her impairment. This will be done by focusing on the identification of feelings and encouraging communication and the use of community resources.

*The texts are noted in parentheses.

Table 1-3 *(cont.)*

Focus of Theory*	Emphasis of Nursing Theory	Clinical Approach
Orlando (*The Dynamic Nurse-Patient Relationship*)	Nursing focuses on meeting patients' immediate needs, which relieves or diminishes their distress or improves their immediate sense of adequacy or well being (p. 5). Patients generally require help when there are physical limitations, when there are adverse reactions to the setting, and when they cannot communicate their needs (p. 11). The nurse's practice centers around observation, reporting, recording, and those actions performed with or for the patient (p. 31).	The immediate need for the patient is having the nurse contact the neighbor. The nurse will then focus on the woman's physical limitations, observe the effect of the emergency room on her reaction, and assist her to communicate her needs.
Hall (*Another View of Nursing Care and Quality*)	Nursing involves the *care* or nurturing of patients, the *core* or therapeutic use of self, and the *cure* of disease with the help of other health care professionals (p. 2). These interrelated aspects differ in their emphasis depending on the patients' present situation and their ability to cope.	Recognizing the woman's feelings about her dog (core), the nurse will contact the neighbor immediately. The nurse, in providing nurturance (care), will also facilitate and carry out the physician's prescription (cure), and assist the woman in coping with her inability to move and face the future. The nurse will focus on the woman's messages about how she feels about her present state and encourage her to make conscious decisions on her own behalf.

Wiedenbach
(*Clinical Nursing—A Helping Art*)

Nursing integrates thoughts, feelings, and overt actions in order to meet a patient's need for help which is set off by a behavioral stimulus, affected by a set of values and beliefs in order to fulfill a specific purpose (p. 11). The major components of practice include philosophy, purpose, practice, and art (p. 12). Practice includes knowledge, judgment, and procedural and communication skills.

The patient's behavior is affected by her beliefs and values relating to her dog and its care. In order to facilitate this care, the nurse calls the neighbor and assures the patient the dog is receiving attention.

The patient's reaction to the nurse and to her immobility will assist the nurse in exploring the patient's ability to resolve her problems. The nurse will administer care to the patient if the plan of care is accepted by the patient.

Levine
(*Introduction to Clinical Nursing*)

Humans respond to the environment holistically. Nursing is based on four conservation principles of energy, structural integrity, personal integrity, and social integrity, which give the rationale for practice (pp. 13–14). Observation, the scientific approach, and communications affect patient-centered nursing interventions.

In order to preserve the patient's social and personal integrity and to facilitate her ability to participate in her care, the nurse will call the neighbor to care for the dog. She will then assess her energy level, her feelings about her wholeness and being immobile, her relationships with others, and her own body's ability to heal structurally.

Johnson
(*Conceptual Models for Nursing Practice*)

A behavioral system includes all the patterned repetitive and purposeful ways of behaving. A highly complex system contains parts or subsystems which can be described and analyzed. Each subsystem has drives and goals, a predisposition to act, a scope of action, and a behavior. They include attachment or affiliative, sexual, eliminative, aggressive/protective, achievement, ingestive, restorative, and dependency subsystems (pp. 207–215). Nurturance, protection, and stimulation of the subsystem are the basis of nursing practice.

The nurse, being aware of the patient's attachment to her dog, will call the neighbor. She will protect and stimulate the mobility of the patient during her care in order to facilitate purposeful ways of behaving and to restore her sense of independence.

Table 1-3 (*cont.*)

Focus of Theory*	Emphasis of Nursing Theory	Clinical Approach
Rogers (*Theoretical Basis of Nursing*)	Nursing's central focus is the study of the unity of man and the process of life, which is expressed in assumptions. Such assumptions include those that man is a unified whole, an open system exchanging energy with the environment, unidirectional with change, having pattern and organization characterized by language and emotion (pp. 41–72). Nursing is concerned with human health and welfare.	Since the patient's energy and environment have an effect on her health and welfare, the nurse will first call the neighbor about the dog. The nurse will then identify the patient's total patterns of behaving, especially in terms of her moving ahead toward health and mobility. Change in the patient's ability to move and become independent will guide care.
Orem (*Nursing: Concepts of Practice*)	Nursing is a human service which focuses on the need for self-care provided by the individual or the nurse in order to sustain life or recover from disease (p. 6). Self-care need requisites are (1) universal, such as the need for air, water, food, (2) related to health deviation, such as changes in extremities or healing, and (3) developmental, such as those related to children and their needs (p. 141).	The nurse identifies the universal self-care requests of maintaining bonds of affection, love, and friendship and allows the patient to call her neighbor and arrange for the dog's care. The nurse will analyze her patient's ability to care for herself in relation to her health deviation needs. Later she will either provide care to meet the deficits or educate the patient to meet her own needs.

King
(A Theory for Nursing: Systems, Concepts, Process)

Nursing is a process involving perceptions, judgments, actions, reactions, interactions, and transactions that lead to a goal attainment. The focus of nursing is related to human beings interacting with their environment in order to achieve health. Health involves human growth and development, adjustment to stresses, and the use of resources within a culture. Personal, interpersonal, and social systems show the relationship among the concepts identified within the theory.

Travelbee
(Interpersonal Aspects of Nursing)

Nursing is an interpersonal process that assists the individual, family, or community to prevent or cope with the stress of illness and suffering or to find meaning in such experiences (p. 7). The interaction involves a human-to-human relationship in order to achieve the goal of nursing. Communication skills and abilities with an underlying theoretical basis of the nature of human beings and the meaning of illness, suffering, and health are essential to practice (p. 97).

The nurse and patient perceive the initial goal as that of meeting the needs of the patient's dog, and the nurse calls the neighbor directly. The interaction between the patient and nurse becomes the focus in terms of the patient's immobility and her ability to further develop and adjust to stresses and use resources available to her. The individual's perception of her body image, her ability to communicate with others, and her fears of loneliness will influence her ability to regain health. The nurse understands that the immediate meaning of illness to this patient is her inability to cope with her dog's needs not being met. Thus, the nurse calls the neighbor and arranges for the care of the dog. Emphasis is placed on effective communication between the nurse and the patient in relationship to the stress of being immobile and the suffering she is experiencing. The nurse will assist the patient in finding some meaning in this illness experience.

Table 1-3 (cont.)

Focus of Theory*	Emphasis of Nursing Theory	Clinical Approach
Neuman (The Neuman System Model)	Nursing is a total person approach in which we view the individual in relationship to stress. The aim is to reduce stress factors and adverse conditions that interfere with wellness by increasing the amount of energy that is stored. Humans have a normal line of defense and resistance to stressors. Nursing identifies the patient's ability to defend or resist such stressors and develops the means to prevent further stress. Stressors occur within, between, and outside the individual (pp. 10–14).	The nurse realizes that the patient has experienced several stressors and has reduced energy with which to deal with her situation. In order to reduce her stress/concern for her dog, she contacts the neighbor and arranges for the pet's care. Emphasis will be placed on preventing further stress in the patient and minimizing her loss of energy due to immobility. The latter concern can be accomplished by improving her lines of defense, such as through exercise and/or rest, and by assisting her in resisting other stressors, such as the feeling of helplessness.
Roy (Theory Construction in Nursing)	Nursing views the person as an adaptive system which reacts to stimuli in four modes. These adaptive modes are related to physiological needs, such as the need for fluids and oxygen, the self-concept, role functioning, and interdependence. Persons experience adaptation problems which need to be minimized in order to allow them to cope with other stimuli and to maintain health (pp. 41–44).	The major initial stimulus that is interfering with the patient's ability to adapt to her condition and the environment of the emergency room is her concern for her dog. This relates to her self-concept, role, and interdependence. Calling her neighbor and reducing the major stimuli will allow the nurse to focus on other stimuli, such as her physiological need for movement and her ability to adapt to immobility.

Kinlein
(*Independent Nursing Practice with Clients*)

The formal objective of nursing is caring for the body, mind, and soul of a person. The focus is the person's health state in relation to his self-care practices and the nurse as a self-care agent. It is through knowledge and experience and the continuous contact with the client that the outcome of care will be more predictable (pp. 15–24).

The nurse recognizes that the patient is immobile and cannot care for herself and her dog. She contacts the neighbor and then proceeds to focus continuously on the patient's ability to care for herself based on her strength (such as her ability to move her left side) and her deficits (such as her inability to walk). She will view the patient as becoming increasingly healthy as she becomes more independent and has greater self-care assets.

Watson
(*Philosophy and Science of Caring*)

The science of caring involves the interpersonal process in relation to meeting certain human needs to promote health and growth of individuals and families through a humanistic altruistic system of values. Faith, hope, and the development of a helping-trust relationship within a supportive, protective, and corrective environment are essential.

The nurse, after realizing that the patient's immediate need is to have her dog cared for, calls the neighbor. This assists the nurse in establishing a supportive-trusting relationship, which includes faith and hope with the patient in relation to her potential, in order to facilitate her health, growth, and development.

In reviewing the clinical situation described in Table 1-3, remember that the nurse may also want to approach nursing care by integrating the themes of more than one theorist. Such an integration might prove helpful in dealing with patients who have multiple problems or needs. For example, the nurse may choose to allow the patient to contact the neighbor in order to assist her in meeting her own needs (Orem), which would also reduce the stimuli and assist her in adapting (Roy), and then focus on her energy level in terms of her physiological needs (Levine) by careful observation and effective communication. The chapters that follow will increasingly demonstrate that there are similarities and differences among the theories within each of the themes and between the major themes, yet the integration of the major ideas is feasible and probably beneficial in practice.

These clinical approaches (Table 1-3) demonstrate the following in relation to the use of theory:

The patient's concern for her dog rather than herself influenced the nurse's *initial* plan of care.

The way in which the nurse *viewed* the total patient and the environment differed with each theoretical approach.

The *focus* of nursing care in dealing with this patient differed more between some theorists than others.

The specific *outcome* of nursing care may or may not differ.

All theories focus on assisting the patient to return to a positive state of wellness or health.

There are many ways of thinking about patients—their needs, their abilities to adapt, the stimuli or stressors they experience, their relationships with others and with the environment, their energy levels. It is no longer adequate to view patients from a medical perspective in relation to technical skills and physicians' medication orders if we are to practice professionally and focus on human beings.

REFERENCES

Abdellah, F.G., I.L. Beland, A. Martin, and R.V. Matheney. *Patient-Centered Approaches to Nursing.* New York: Macmillan, Inc., 1960.

Hall, L.E. "Another View of Nursing Care and Quality." In *Continuity of Patient Care: The Role of Nursing,* edited by K.M. Straub and K.S. Parker, pp. 47–60. Washington, D.C.: Catholic University Press, 1966.

Harmer, B., and V. Henderson. *Textbook of Principles and Practice of Nursing*, 5th ed. New York: Macmillan, Inc., 1955.

Johnson, D.E. "The Behavioral System For Nursing." In *Conceptual Models for Nursing Practice*, 2d ed., edited by J.P. Riehl and Sr. C. Roy. New York: Appleton-Century-Crofts, 1980, pp. 207–216.

King, I.M. *A Theory of Nursing: Systems, Concepts, Process.* New York: John Wiley & Sons, Inc., 1981.

Kinlein, M.L. *Independent Nursing Practice and Clients.* Philadelphia: J.B. Lippincott, 1977.

Levine, M.E. *Introduction to Clinical Nursing*, 2d ed. Philadelphia: F.A. Davis Company, 1973.

Neuman, B. *The Neuman Systems Model: Application to Nursing Education and Practice.* East Norwalk, Conn.: Appleton-Century-Crofts, 1982.

Nightingale, F. *Notes on Nursing: What It Is and What It Is Not.* New York: Dover Publications, Inc., 1969. (Unabridged republication of the first American edition, as published in 1860 by D. Appleton & Company.)

Orem, D.E. *Nursing: Concepts of Practice.* New York: McGraw-Hill Book Company, 1971.

Orlando, I.J. *The Dynamic Nurse-Patient Relationship: Function, Process, and Principles.* New York: G.P. Putnam's Sons, 1961.

Peplau, H.E. *Interpersonal Relations in Nursing.* New York: G.P. Putnam's Sons, 1952.

Rogers, M.E. *An Introduction to the Theoretical Basis of Nursing.* Philadelphia: F.A. Davis Company, 1970.

Roy, C., and S. Roberts. *Theory Construction in Nursing: An Adaptation Model.* Englewood Cliffs, N.J.: Prentice-Hall, Inc., 1981.

Travelbee, J. *Interpersonal Aspects of Nursing*, 2d ed. Philadelphia: F.A. Davis Company, 1971.

Watson, J. *Nursing: The Philosophy and Science of Caring.* Boston: Little, Brown & Company, 1979.

Wiedenbach, E. *Clinical Nursing: A Helping Art.* New York: Springer Publishing Company, Inc., 1964.

2

THE MEANING OF THEORY

INTRODUCTION

In order to be able to practice nursing with a theoretical approach, it is essential to have an understanding of the development and meaning of theory. Nursing theories basically give us ideas about the way we look at nursing situations in order to achieve certain goals. We must understand the relative merit of a particular theory for practice so that we can become aware of its potential impact on nursing care.

The meaning of the word *theory* varies both among professional disciplines and within the disciplines themselves. We have already been exposed to many theories—biological theories about the function of cells, psychological theories about how children develop, sociological theories about the family, and political theories about government's impact on our lives. In order to understand any scientific or professional field, we must understand the theories that are basic to the discipline. Although each of these disciplines would claim to have theories, the meaning, purpose, and use of such theories is controversial; this is also presently true in nursing.

THE FUNCTIONS OF THEORY

Theory can offer four functions to nursing practice: *describing, explaining, predicting,* and *controlling practice.** Theory organizes the relationships between the complex events that occur in a nursing situation so that we can assist human beings. Simply stated, *theory provides a way of thinking about and looking at the world around us.*

In order to view and explain the world, we need to use words when we communicate or think. When we use words, we need to understand their real meanings to us. Such meanings are often based on what we know or assume, and often differ from one person to another. Our words also have relationships to each other. One word must be used to define another. Dictionaries often list multiple definitions of the same word, and the definitions are frequently circular—one word means another word which means another and often leads us back to the first word we looked up. For example, *to assist* means *to help—to help* means *to assist.* When we define words in a certain way and find relationships between different words or among similar words, we are often making assumptions. Such assumptions frequently lead us to develop statements that explain our world to us. When we think logically, we go through this process in order to come to some conclusions that lead us to behave in a certain way. Loosely speaking, we are theorizing or speculating constantly.

In looking at Table 2-1 in terms of the basic components and meanings of theory, you can see that the path taken to develop theory is similar to the process through which we form our everyday speculations about the world and how we fit into it. The words are really *concepts,* the meanings are our definitions of the words, our

Table 2-1

Components of Theory

Terminology	Basic Meaning
Concepts	Word or words
Definitions	Meaning
Models	Outline/assumptions
Propositions	Sentences and relationship to statements
Theory	Descriptive, explanatory
	Predictive and control statements

*A useful text to further understand theory as it relates to nursing is: Chinn, P., and M.K. Jacobs *Theory and Nursing: A Systematic Approach.* St. Louis: The C.V. Mosby Company, 1983.

assumptions reflect some image or *model,* and the assumptions lead to some type of relationships, which are *propositions.* We speak in sentences relating one word to another. When we do so to describe or explain our view of the world, we take a theoretical approach. This meaning of theory which is noted in Table 2-1 could also include a vision that we have about the world as well as a law or fact that is truly valid based on research.

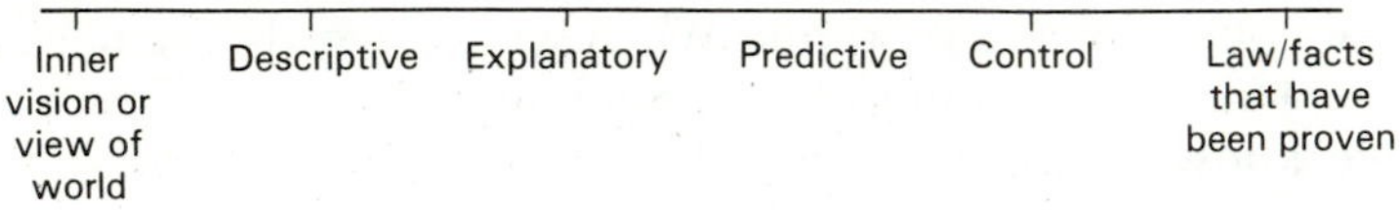

Inner vision or view of world	Descriptive	Explanatory	Predictive	Control	Law/facts that have been proven

Figure 2-1. Theory continuum.

The theory continuum is not finite but is merely a way of viewing how we move along mentally from one level of thinking about theory to another. We all relate to others and to the world around us from our own inner view or vision of the world. At times, we make a great effort to describe what we see or feel and how we interpret events based on our perceptions. We explain our behavior based on such descriptions, and it is not uncommon for us to predict what will happen based on those descriptions. In our personal lives, dealing on the level of vision and description is adequate and functional. For professionals who must behave based on expected results, however, theory needs to be at least explanatory if not predictive.

CONCEPTS

A nursing theory, as other theories do, has multiple components that lead to its development (Table 2-2). These components are *concepts.* Even the word *concept* requires a definition and the identification of characteristics for clarity, since it is also a concept. *Concepts are images that describe objects, properties, or events and give meaning to our perceptions.* We perceive things by developing mental pictures of something that is probably not present in the environment. Members of a particular group, such as nurses, tend to have similar mental pictures based on their common attitude and orientation toward a particular concept.

When nurses in a hospital communicate about the concept *bed,* they tend to think of the typical hospital bed that can be raised and lowered to enable the patient to get out of bed when it is in the lower position and to enable nurses to care for the patient when the bed is in the higher position. If a group of army recruits were told that their *beds* were in a particular building, they might think about

Table 2-2

Model for Nursing Theory

Components of Theory	Definition of Terms	Nursing Theory
Concepts	Images that describe objects, properties, or events and give meaning to our perception	Human/Environment/ Health/Nursing
Definitions	Criteria and characteristics of the concepts	Definition of concepts within theory. For example, humans have biological, psychological, and ecological needs.
Models	Diagrammatic—outline/ structural design	Humans—Environment $\times$ Health—Nursing
Propositions	An expression of relationships offered for consideration or acceptance	*Nursing* influences the impact of the *environment* on the *individual's health status.*
Theory	Organizes the relationship among the concepts to describe, explain, predict, and control practice	*Description*—The patient/ client situation is represented in such a way as to give a focus to the practice of nursing. *Explanation*—There is a logical relationship between the events with a client and situation that influences the impact of nursing care on the individual. *Prediction*—Given certain approaches to nursing care, one can foretell the outcomes based on scientific reasoning. *Control*—Theory can be used to produce a desired outcome.

army cots. Many potential images can come to mind when we think of something as concrete as *bed.* A double bed, a hide-a-bed, and a folding bed are just some possibilities. All these images relating to the concept *bed* refer to something we can sleep on. We also use the concept *bed* to refer to a flat or level surface, such as a plot of ground prepared for plants. There is a commonality between the use of the concept *bed* for something we lie on and sleep in and a flat surface for seeds to rest on: Both relate to a flat surface.

The Concept Continuum:
Empirical to Abstract

The concept *bed* as an object is basically *empirical.* Through experience and observation, we can count the number of beds in a room at a given point in time. The concept bed is a reliable indicator if we want to identify the bedroom within the house. Thus, empirical concepts

1. are absolute and reliable indications.
2. stand unequivocally distinguishable from and exclusive of other concepts.
3. are fixed at a given point in time.
4. need fewer criteria or identified characteristics for clarity.

Examples of empirical concepts are *male, Oriental, income,* and *thirty-three years old.* Each of these is relatively absolute, is clearly distinguishable from other concepts at a given moment, and needs little real explanation for two individuals to perceive like imagery.

Concepts are said to be more *abstract* when it is more difficult for different persons to perceive the same thing. Such concepts have more generality and are more related to an event or property. Concepts such as health, love, and nursing have few specific criteria or characteristics to describe their meaning, and specific criteria are difficult to develop.

Concepts not only range from empirical (male) to abstract (love), but they can also fall anywhere between these two points, depending on our ability to perceive similar images when thinking about them. The more our images differ or are questionable, the more *abstract* the concept will be. The more we can directly observe or experience the concept, the more *empirical* the concept will be. In nursing we can often indirectly observe such concepts as blood pressure or temperature by using instruments to measure them. We do not specifically have an image of a temperature; we relate it to a person's condition. This concept may be said to be understood by *inference.*

Different sciences tend to have certain types of concepts. Chemistry, biology, and medical science tend to deal with more empirical concepts than nursing or the behavioral sciences do.

Table 2-3 gives examples of concepts that are more empirical or more abstract and identifies how we generally define the concept in a particular case.

Table 2-3

Empirical (directly observable)	Inference (indirectly observable)	Abstract (indirectly observable)
Specific age	Pain	Empathy
Gender	Family	Prejudice
Home address	Temperature	Personality
Anatomical parts	X ray	Caring
		Fear
Physical assessment data	Laboratory reports	Psychosocial assessment data

In gathering data the physician will deal with both directly observable and inferential types of concepts. The physical examination is basically a biological review of the patient, which is the empirical evidence that the physician uses in order to decide what additional data are essential. The use of laboratory reports and X rays, which are not directly observed but imply a certain biological status, will also assist in the diagnosis of disease. Nursing does use this information for practice, but it goes beyond the empirical to deal with more abstract concepts like fear, empathy, and anxiety. These are nonobservable and need specific criteria if someone is to understand their meaning. Utilizing such abstract concepts also creates more difficulty in finding meaning in nursing theories. The development of nursing theories, like the development of psychological theories, requires the use of concepts that cannot be easily and directly observed and researched from a biological perspective.

In Table 2-2, note that the basic concepts that are included, in some way, in all nursing theories are *human, environment, health,* and *nursing* (Torres and Yura, 1974). All of these concepts are abstract and require the identification of specific criteria in order to make them functional within a given nursing theory. For example, the environment as described by Florence Nightingale is related to water, air, noise, and smell. To Martha Rogers it describes the human energy field. In the discussion of the nursing theories throughout the book, the use and meaning of these four concepts within each of the theories will be reviewed.

MODELS

In order to give some meaning to the relationships between the concepts, *models* are developed. This helps us visualize diagrammatically how one concept influences and logically or causally connects with

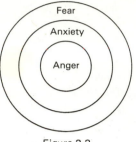

Figure 2-2.

another. An example of a core identification model is shown in Figure 2-2.

Within this model *anger,* is viewed as central or core to *anxiety* and *fear. Fear* encompasses *anxiety* and *anger.*

Utilizing the three concepts of fear, anxiety, and anger, a nondirectional model would look like Figure 2-3. Here, there is a relationship between *fear* and *anger, anger* and *anxiety,* and *fear* and *anxiety;* which concept is central or which concept leads to the other is unclear.

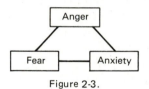

Figure 2-3.

The three concepts—*anger, fear,* and *anxiety*—are foundational when they are arranged as shown in Figure 2-4.

Figure 2-4.

Fear is basic to *anxiety,* and both *anxiety* and *fear* are basic to *anger.*

In approaching the linear-directional model of the concepts of *anger, fear,* and *anxiety,* the model would look like Figure 2-5.

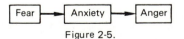

Figure 2-5.

A circular model of the concepts of *fear, anxiety,* and *anger* would appear as shown in Figure 2-6.

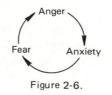

Figure 2-6.

Figure 2-7 gives some examples of how one could model the components of theory to show their relationships. Different models

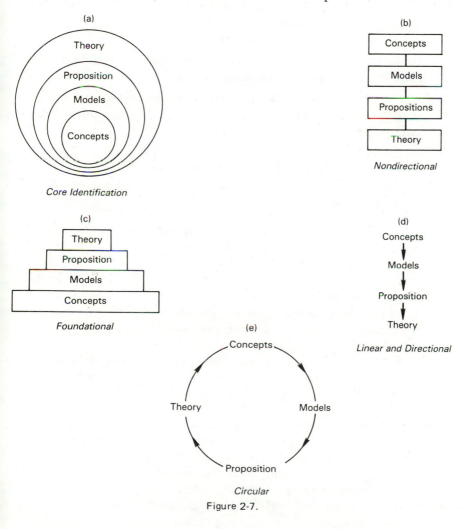

Figure 2-7.

help explain how one thinks of or imagines the connection between each component. The following statements can be inferred and assumed from each model:

Model A—Core identification: The concepts are central to the entire development of the theory. They are included in all the other components of theory. Models include concepts but concepts do *not* include models, propositions, or theory. Theory includes all the other components.

Model B—Nondirectional: The four components of theory are related sequentially to one another. Concepts relate to models, models to propositions, and propositions to theory. The relationship between concept, model, and theory is not a direct but an indirect one, through a proposition.

Model C—Foundational: Concepts are viewed as foundational to models, models basic to propositions, and so on.

Model D—Linear and directional: Concepts lead to models, models lead to concepts and propositions, and propositions lead only to theory.

Model E—Circular: At any given point each of the components leads sequentially to the next component. Theory could lead to the identification and clarification of a concept, particularly an abstract one.

All of the models are valid and are based on some common assumptions about theory analysis and development.

1. In order to develop or understand theories, we must deal with concepts.
2. Models relate to concepts and propositions.
3. Propositions relate to models and theory.

In Table 2-2, the four basic concepts of nursing theories (human, environment, health, and nursing) are modeled in such a way as to show that there is a relationship between each. Humans relate to health, nursing, and the environment; nursing to health, environment, and humans; and so forth. It is possible to create other models based on different assumptions. For an example, review Figure 2-8.

The assumptions in this model are that nursing relates to the environment, which surrounds humans. The environment, which encompasses humans, relates to nursing and health. The *only* relationship between nursing and health is through the environment. Humans

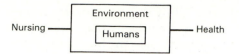

Figure 2-8. From: Gertrude Torres, "Florence Nightingale", Julia B. George, "Lydia E. Hall", in *NURSING THEORIES: The Base for Professional Nursing Practice,* 2nd Ed., edited by Julia B. George, © 1985, pp. 41, 115. Reprinted by permission of Prentice-Hall, Inc., Englewood Cliffs, N.J.

do *not* have a direct relationship with nursing and health. The question as to whether these assumptions are true or not is not important at this point. Models merely help us think about concepts in different ways. Many nurse-theorists use models to explain the relationship between the concepts they use. It should be noted that models may be used in combination by various theorists; one can, for example, integrate the core and circular model. You will note this in the following chapters.

PROPOSITIONS

The above assumptions are expressions of relationships that are possible within the model. These are called *propositions.* Propositions (also called *assumptions*) are basically unstable and can be found to be false in the future, usually by research. They are developed as proposals to be considered for acceptance as truth.

In Table 2-2, the proposition "nursing influences the impact of the environment on the individual's health status" evolves from the model. This statement offers for consideration a way of viewing nursing. Within their theories, nursing theorists offer propositions that have implications for nursing practice. These theories should be considered for testing to determine their truthfulness.

In the development of propositions, statements are made that show specific types of relationships among the concepts. For example, consider the abstract concepts *violence* and *poverty* in terms of the following propositions:

If there is poverty, there will be violence.

If there is violence, there will be poverty.

If there is poverty, there is always violence.

Violence and poverty occur at the same time.

Poverty is necessary for violence to occur.

To some readers, all of these assumptions seem to be truths. To others, one or more may seem to be inaccurate in relation to observation and experiences. One basic problem in making such decisions at this point is that the abstract concepts have not been clearly defined, so the proposition has different meanings to us. What is poverty? A family income below $5000 or $20,000 a year? What is violence? Pushing someone out of your way or killing someone? It is only when there is a clear definition of the concepts that the proposition can be stated with clarity and used for research.

THEORY

Theory development is the identification of a proposition that has not been shown to be false with continued research. It is difficult to show that a proposition is true because it is usually impossible to test every instance or case relating to a particular proposition. As long as the proposition is repeatedly studied through research and found never to be false, we can continue to believe it to be true. Such propositions within a given theory will describe or predict nursing action (Table 2-2). For example, consider the situation of a seventy-year-old patient who has refused to eat the evening meal in the nursing home dining room. A theory that helps describe the situation might assist the nurse in focusing on the patient's perception, which, combined with the nurse's perception, observation, and experiences, would assist the nurse in sharing the data received from the patient with other nurses in order to help the patient. If the theory were to explain the relationship between different events within that situation, the impact of certain actions would be better understood, and the most appropriate plan of care could be identified. If certain events or perceptions were present in this situation, and if the nurse could foretell the outcome of a particular approach, the theory would be predictive in nature. The theory that could control the situation might be ideal. Any theoretical approach is of assistance to the nurse, but a theory that can predict outcomes is most useful. To date, most nursing theories are descriptive, some are explanatory, but none is truly predictive.

Evaluation of Theory

The usefulness of nursing theory is based on an evaluation of its effect on practice. A theory with poorly defined concepts cannot be very useful. Well-defined concepts with illogical relationships are also not helpful. Each component of the theory must be well developed in order for the theory to be useful for practice. Table 2-4 gives the criteria for evaluation of each component. At this time, no nursing or health-related theory meets all the criteria very well. They all have strengths and weaknesses and must be viewed with that in mind. As more and more research is carried out in relation to specific nursing theories, nursing knowledge will become increasingly sophisticated.

Table 2-4

Evaluation of Theory

Components of Theory	Evaluation Criteria
Concepts and definitions	Relate to the basic concepts of nursing
	Are clearly defined with specific criteria/characteristics
	Empirical and/or abstract concepts are easily identified
	Stated with economy of words
	Free from vagueness and ambiguity (uncertainty/indistinctness
	Identify whether certain concepts are ranked/hierarchical in nature
	Defined consistently within the theory
Models	Show logical relationship between concepts
	Are simple rather than complex in their presentation
	Utilize only the relevant concepts from the theory
	Show clear relationships between objects, properties, and events
Propositions	Explain the relationship between the concepts
	Are verifiable so that data can be collected to disprove them
	Are congruent with existing knowledge
	Stay within appropriate limitations
Theory	Can describe, explain, predict, and control intended outcomes and goals for practice.
	Can generate other theories by describing new relationships between concepts

Evaluation of Concepts

The definition, evaluation, and analysis of concepts, especially those that are abstract, are difficult and time consuming. In attempting to clearly define a concept, we develop criteria/characteristics that often explain other concepts as well. For example, the concept *empathy* is frequently used in nursing but often is not well understood. *Related* concepts are sympathy, pity, and compassion (Forsyth, 1980, p. 38), according to Forsyth, who has developed essential criteria that differentiate empathy from the related concepts. All four concepts contain consciousness, temporality (the here and now), relationship, and intensity. Empathy involves accuracy of perception, validation of experiences, objectivity, and freedom from judgment or evaluation. Such criteria represent conditions that must be present in order for empathy to occur. For example, empathy does not include subjective involvement with the feelings of another, since that places one in the position of also needing help. Empathy is not demeaning like pity, or sorrowful like compassion. There are also concepts that are *contrary* to the concept empathy. Advice giving and superficiality in a relationship are certainly instances when empathy is not present. Sometimes identifying what we know is *not* the criterion for a specific concept can be helpful. We know that disease and pain are not criteria for health. A related concept to health is wellness or well-being. Thus, in the development of criteria to clarify specific concepts, we need to review *related* and *contrary* concepts so that we can differentiate the meaning.

Evaluation of Models

Models must reflect the major concepts within a given theory. If concepts are added or ignored, the propositions that follow will be incomplete and inaccurate. As noted in Figure 2-3 (relating to the components of the theory) various models are possible, each offering a somewhat different relationship between the concepts (in this case the concepts are the components of the theory). Some relationships between concepts appear more logical and valid than others. For example, the relationship between the two concepts *unemployment* and *social isolation* is, for the most part, obvious, so a line could be drawn between them in a model. It is less appropriate to directly connect the concepts *starvation* and *well-being.*

Models should be relatively easy to follow, rather simple in their presentation, and easily understood. The relationship between the concepts should be so clearly developed that anyone would be able to state the same propositions. The model shown in Figure 2-9, which is circular, linear, and directional, is offered by Bigbee (1983, p. 158) relating to adolescent obesity. The emphasis is on the *locus of control* in adolescent obesity. Locus of control relates to the individual's perception as to whether one is controlled by external or internal forces. Internal control is the individual's perception that his behavior is most influential in terms of an outcome; external control reflects the belief that outside forces affect the outcome. (A *paradigm* integrates multiple theories.)

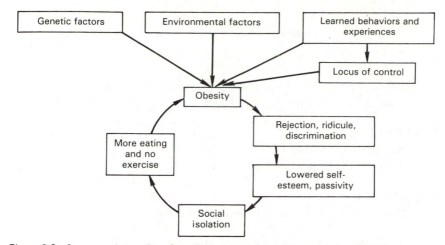

Figure 2-9. Conceptual paradigm for adolescent obesity from *Advances in Nursing Theory Development*, edited by Chinn, Figure 9-1, p. 158, © 1983. Reprinted with permission of Aspen Systems Corporation.

Within the model shown in Figure 2-9, there are four forces noted in a linear manner which influence obesity—genetic factors, environmental factors, learned behaviors and experiences, and locus of control. Also note that learned behaviors and experiences influence locus of control. Within the circular section of this model we see that obesity leads to rejection, which leads to lowered self-esteem, which leads to social isolation, which leads to more eating, which again leads to obesity. The relationships among the concepts are clear, so that propositions can be developed. Are the following propositions valid for the model?

Ridicule will lead to passivity.

Environment factors affect obesity.

Lowered self-esteem leads to social isolation.

All are correct, and many more could be developed from this model.

Evaluation of Propositions

Propositions that are well stated can be used to develop research statements. Thus, data/information can be collected in order to verify that in any particular situation the proposition remains true and the

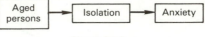

Figure 2-10.

concepts do have a particular relationship. For example, review the linear and directional model in Figure 2-10.

Valid Propositions
　　A. Age leads to isolation and anxiety.
　　B. Anxiety stems from isolation as humans age.

Inappropriate Proposition
　　C. Anxiety of the aged is caused by isolation.

Propositions A and B stay within the appropriate limits of the model. The relationship between the three concepts—aged person, isolation, and anxiety—flow from one to the other. Proposition C implies that isolation of the aging is the only cause for anxiety. Data collected showing that anxiety that is not related to isolation exists among the aged would demonstrate that the proposition is false. For example, in studying preoperative aged clients in the hospital, fear of surgery and pain, and *not* a sense of isolation, may be the cause of anxiety at that time.

With continued research and verification of the relationships between the concepts, theories will develop that will either describe the relationship between isolation and anxiety among the aged, explain the relationship of these concepts, or predict the outcomes of isolation of the aged and control the outcomes. Thus we will have developed theory for practice.

REFERENCES

Bigbee, J. "Locus of Control and the Obese Adolescent: A Pilot Study." In *Advances in Nursing Theory Development,* edited by P.L. Chinn. Maryland: Aspen, 1983.

Chinn, P., and M. Jacobs. *Theory and Nursing: A Systematic Approach.* St. Louis, Mo.: The C.V. Mosby Company, 1983.

Forsyth, G. F. "Analysis of Concept of Empathy: Illustration of One Approach." *Advances in Nursing Science.* Vol. 2, no. 2, January 1980.

3

NURSING THEORY
AND NURSING PROCESS

INTRODUCTION

Theory is knowledge that is used for practice, while *process* is the method used to apply theory. *Theory* is the content; *process* is the way of using that content. Theory contains concepts that are related in such a way as to describe, explain, or predict events, while process is the method of thinking about theory. The use of the words *theory* and *process* in nursing are similar to the use of the words *science* and *art*. *Science* and *theory* represent the theoretical base for practice, while *process* and *art* reflect the skill of nursing practice. *Skills* are the ability to use theoretical knowledge effectively in practice. Intellectual skills such as critical thinking or decision making are as important as, or perhaps more important than, technical skills.

The integration of theory and process is the basis for professional nursing practice. One cannot function without the other. It is impossible to provide nursing care without processing knowledge in some way. Neither theory nor process is instinctive; both must be learned. In other words, we are not born knowing, nor do our life experiences adequately explain, how to appropriately process knowledge in nursing.

PROCESS

The word *process* means *to advance* by gradually changing something so that a particular result will occur. Thus the nursing process is a method used by professional nurses to change a client situation for a specific goal. Involved in the nursing process is a continuous modification of goals and evaluation of progress.

Lawyers, computer scientists, and photographers use different processes in order to achieve particular goals. Each must learn both the theory of their field and the way of processing that theory. Regardless of the method used, all involve a sequence of events and a procedure for handling the knowledge or theory. The following steps are usually used:

1. Gathering of specific information related to a life event
2. Application of knowledge to the particular situation
3. Analysis of information in relation to knowledge
4. Development of a plan(s) to achieve a goal(s)
5. Continuation of behavior/action
6. Assessment of progress

A systematic approach to change is represented here. Although the steps appear linear and sequential, in reality no clear demarcation exists. For example, additional information is constantly being gathered during each of the other steps, especially during the planned behavior/action.

The gathering of information and the application of knowledge direct the entire process. They are foundational or basic to any plan, goal, or action. If inadequate or inaccurate information is obtained, there can be no appropriate plans or actions. This point must be emphasized: Goals cannot be achieved nor appropriate actions taken unless an accurate theoretical base has been used.

Standards of Practice and the Nursing Process

Table 3-1 shows the *Standards of Nursing Practice,* published by the American Nurses' Association, the professional association for nurses. It provides a systematic approach to nursing practice and reflects nursing's systematic approach to change. There are seven standards, each specifying a rationale and assessment factors. The

Table 3-1

American Nurses' Association Standards of Nursing Practice

STANDARD I

THE COLLECTION OF DATA ABOUT THE HEALTH STATUS OF THE CLIENT/ PATIENT IS SYSTEMATIC AND CONTINUOUS. THE DATA ARE ACCESSIBLE, COM- MUNICATED, AND RECORDED.

Rationale: Comprehensive care requires complete and ongoing collection of data about the client/patient to determine the nursing care needs of the client/patient. All health status data about the client/patient must be available for all members of the health care team.

STANDARD II

NURSING DIAGNOSES ARE DERIVED FROM HEALTH STATUS DATA.

Rationale: The health status of the client/patient is the basis for determining the nursing care needs. The data are analyzed and compared to norms when possible.

STANDARD III

THE PLAN OF NURSING CARE INCLUDES GOALS DERIVED FROM THE NURSING DIAGNOSES.

Rationale: The determination of the results to be achieved is an essential part of planning care.

STANDARD IV

THE PLAN OF NURSING CARE INCLUDES PRIORITIES AND THE PRE- SCRIBED NURSING APPROACHES OR MEASURES TO ACHIEVE THE GOALS DE- RIVED FROM THE NURSING DIAGNOSES.

Rationale: Nursing actions are planned to promote, maintain, and restore the client's/ patient's well-being.

STANDARD V

NURSING ACTIONS PROVIDE FOR CLIENT/PATIENT PARTICIPATION IN HEALTH PROMOTION, MAINTENANCE, AND RESTORATION.

Rationale: The client/patient and family are continually involved in nursing care.

STANDARD VI

NURSING ACTIONS ASSIST THE CLIENT/PATIENT TO MAXIMIZE HIS HEALTH CAPABILITIES.

Rationale: Nursing actions are designed to promote, maintain, and restore health.

STANDARD VII

THE CLIENT'S/PATIENT'S PROGRESS OR LACK OF PROGRESS TOWARD GOAL ACHIEVEMENT IS DETERMINED BY THE CLIENT/PATIENT AND THE NURSE.

Rationale: The quality of nursing care depends upon comprehensive and intelligent deter- mination of nursing's impact upon the health status of the client/patient. The client/pa- tient is an essential part of this determination.

STANDARD VIII

THE CLIENT'S/PATIENT'S PROGRESS OR LACK OF PROGRESS TOWARD GOAL ACHIEVEMENT DIRECTS REASSESSMENT, REORDERING OF PRIORITIES, NEW GOAL SETTING, AND REVISION OF THE PLAN OF NURSING CARE.

Rationale: The nursing process remains the same, but the input of new information may dic- tate new or revised approaches.

From *Standards of Nursing Practice*, ANA, Kansas City, Missouri.

Table 3-2

ANA Standards	Steps of Nursing Process
I. Collection of data	Assessment—gather information about the health status of a client/patient.
II. Nursing diagnosis	Nursing diagnosis—statement of the health status of the client/patient based on an analysis of the data.
III. Plans and goals IV. Identify priorities and measures to achieve a goal	Plans—organized statement of action needed to achieve goal.
V. Client/patient participation in nursing actions VI. Actions assist client/patient to maximize health capabilities	Implementation—the action dictated by the information, health status, and goals of the client/patient and/or nurse.
VII. Data to identify progress toward goal VIII. Reordering of priorities and goals	Evaluation—the reanalysis of the health status of the client in relation to the achieved goals.

standards offer the nurse a way to view the quality of nursing care and incorporate the nursing process, as noted in Table 3-2.

As noted in Table 3-2 the nursing process is usually viewed as having five steps, while the *Standards of Practice* incorporates eight standards. Some of the literature offers four steps to the nursing process, integrating assessment and nursing diagnosis into one. Some of the content in the *Standards of Practice* is basically similar to the steps of the nursing process. This text will utilize the five steps of the nursing process while incorporating all the ideas from the *Standards of Nursing Practice.*

The use of nursing theories within the steps of the nursing process is foundational to practice within the Standards. Particular statements reflect the focus on different nursing theories; note Table 3-3.

Table 3-3

Statements within Standards	Particular Nursing Theories and Focus
Assessment of interactive patterns	Peplau—interpersonal relation
Assessment of environment	Nightingale—proper environment facilitates health
Client/patient capabilities and limitations	Orem—assist in the self-care needs of the client/patient
Client/patient perception of health status	King—nursing involves the perception of the client/patient in relation to the goal of nursing care.
Biophysical status	Henderson and Abdellah—emphasis is placed on meeting the biophysical needs or problems encountered during illness.

Within the Standards, the emphasis is on comprehensive nursing care. This rather complete or broad approach to nursing takes, for example, the client's biological, psychological, sociological, spiritual, and environmental needs, health, illness, family, and resources into account. Thus, any of the nursing theories, in combination or individually, can be used with the Standards. The content, knowledge, or framework for viewing the situation is through nursing theories, and the scientific process of decision making is through the use of the Standards/nursing process.

It is important to realize that the nursing process and the use of a nursing theoretical approach is *unique* to the profession or discipline of nursing. Although, as stated previously, many professionals use a process to solve problems or plan a course of action, the combination of nursing theories and the focus of nursing on health and human beings within the environment is distinct. Certain assumptions follow this way of approaching nursing.

Nursing complements but is distinct from medicine in its use of theoretical content such as nursing theories. Nursing, rather than using the pathological orientation of disease as its emphasis, assists the patient by using a comprehensive, total view of the individual. This will become increasingly clear with a greater understanding and use of nursing theories for practice. In reviewing the standards of care we see that the problems or needs created by an individual's illness or disease process are the focus, not the disease itself.

The Steps of the Process

The nursing process is not really a linear process; its five major steps have been modeled in many ways. One way to view the process is via a directional-linear feedback method, as shown in Figure 3-1.

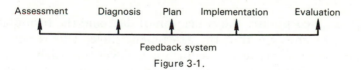

Figure 3-1.

With this approach, following the initial assessment step, evaluation is constantly taking place within the framework of the other four steps. For example, in order to determine whether a teaching plan is effective for a patient who is on a special diet, reassessment, rediagnosis, a revised plan, and a differing approach to the implementation will follow until the patient needs no further teaching or information. New data or information is continuously being gathered while the nurse interacts with the patient, which in turn modifies the nurse's approach.

Another model, which is mostly circular with a core identification, is offered by Jones (1979, p. 69) and is shown in Figure 3-2.

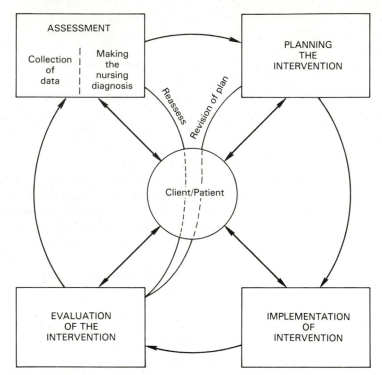

Figure 3-2. The nursing process for the definition of nursing diagnoses. Reprinted with permission from Aspen Systems Corporation, from *Advances in Nursing Science*, 2:1 (October 1979), Figure 1, p. 69.

Jones incorporates the collection of data and the formulation of a nursing diagnosis within the assessment stage. This is not uncommon among other writers. The author believes that each stage of the nursing process as noted in the model moves in a circular manner with the client/patient being in the core. (Here is the combination of the circular and core model.) Also within the model is a feedback system common to the linear model shown in Figure 3-1. Each stage returns to the center—the client—and includes revision after the initial evaluation. Both these models provide for a similar frame of reference or way of thinking about the nursing process. Examples of the use of the nursing process are not presented here since it is theory and process that facilitate nursing care. Thus, in reviewing the nurse theorists later, you will need to review this process in light of the specific nursing theory presented.

It is essential to realize that a medical diagnosis is very different from, as well as inappropriate to use as, a nursing diagnosis. For example, a patient who has had surgery and is complaining of discomfort might have a medical diagnosis of appendicitis and a nursing diagnosis related to pain and its effect. One can see that it is the nursing diagnosis that directs the nurse to administer a pain medication, not the medical diagnosis.

Nursing does have a unique body of theoretical knowledge and a way of processing it which must be learned in order to practice professionally. It is essential for all professionals to think theoretically in their fields, for it is that knowledge that society recognizes as essential for its benefit and care. Many individuals, including nurse's aids and practical nurses, claim to nurse, but unless they can utilize the *Standards of Practice* within the framework of the nursing process and apply specific knowledge, they are not practicing professional nursing or nursing in general. Such nurses are viewed as supportive to the professional nurse, who directs professional care.

High levels of thinking skills, such as analysis, which is appropriate to decision making, are needed to practice nursing. Creative thinking is also required in order to integrate and synthesize various nursing theories in a particular patient situation.

REFERENCES

American Nurses' Association. *Standards of Nursing Practice.* Kansas City: American Nurses' Association, 1973.

Jones, P. "A Terminology for Nursing Diagnoses." In *Advances in Nursing Science* (October 1979), p. 69.

4

ENVIRONMENTAL THEORY

INTRODUCTION

Although many nursing theories explain the relationship between the individual and the environment, as you will see in future chapters, none places as much emphasis on the environment as *Florence Nightingale's*. Nightingale's writing, which describes and explains the role and function of nursing, is the first nursing theory and the only identifiable one between 1860 and 1952. Nightingale's basic theory is written in *Notes on Nursing: What It Is and What It Is Not*. This theory is characteristic of other theories in this book in the following ways:

1. It describes nursing as a discipline that is different from the discipline of medicine.
2. It provides major concepts that assist in describing or explaining the focus of nursing/frame of reference.
3. The relationships between the concepts facilitate the development of a model so that propositions can be identified.
4. The theory can be incorporated into the nursing process so that improved nursing care can be facilitated.

Nightingale's writing preceded most of the scientific theories (such as germ theory), so that her theory is based on the logic and common sense that emerged from her own experiences, especially during the Crimean War. It might be postulated that many of the emerging themes, such as those related to air and water pollution and sleep, stem from some of her ideas.

FLORENCE NIGHTINGALE: DESCRIPTION OF THE THEORY

Frame of reference: $\boxed{\text{human}}$ interact $\boxed{\text{environment}}$

The major concept within her theory is the *environment*, viewed from a physical standpoint. She describes the health of houses and identifies five essential points: pure air, pure water, efficient drainage, cleanliness, and light. A house is unhealthy in proportion to the deficiencies that can be noted among the five points. Pure air basically relates to bringing fresh air into the house to prevent stagnation. Pure water reduces epidemic diseases which were caused by using water polluted by the drainage of sewers and water closets. Efficient drainage requires an untrapped drainage pipe that was outside the walls of the house. Cleanliness is viewed as essential to the prevention of disease. Lighting represents the need for sunlight and fresh outdoor air that is available through open windows. Most of the emphasis is on reducing disease rather than on providing comfort; thus the environment basically encompasses the notion of a clean, well-ventilated and lighted home that has appropriate plumbing—clean water and sewage.

Nursing is not viewed as limited to administering medications and applying poultices, but as oriented toward providing fresh air, light, warmth, cleanliness, quiet, and the proper selection and administration of diet—all at the least expense of vital powers to the patient. Nursing is basically seen as a way of facilitating nature's reparative process by placing the patients in the best condition for nature to act upon them. Nightingale believed that nature alone cures; medicine is the surgery of functions dealing with limbs, organs, and is not curative.

Health is placed in the framework of preventing mostly epidemic diseases and facilitating individuals' ability to heal themselves when disease occurs. In essence, health may be viewed as the absence of disease. *Humans* are also described as those who are with or without disease, and who require a proper environment to achieve health.

Models of Nightingale's Theory

Utilizing the four major concepts in nursing, a model of Nightingale's theory evolves, as shown in Figure 4-1.

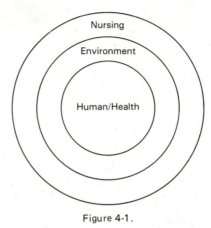

Figure 4-1.

This *core* identification model places *human/health* in the center as the focus or goal of the theory which is strongly influenced by the *environment*. *Nursing* surrounds the other concepts and most immediately the environment of the human and the health of the environment. The reason that *human* and *health* are within the center of the core together, rather than having *human* separated and central, and *health* outside circling *human*, is that within this theory, humans are not discussed, for the most part, except in relation to their health state.

The propositions that emerge from the model are the following:

Nursing is related to the environment of the individual.

The individual's health is related to his environment.

Nursing relates to the health of the individual through its relationship with the environment.

A more detailed model can be developed that would incorporate the characteristics of the theory (Figure 4-2). Again, the nurse's role is mostly to modify the physical environment which affects the human being and his state of health. Within the physical environment, air is the first essential upon which all the rest depends. This is consistent with need theories developed later, as you will note in the next chapter.

Nightingale provided many propositions/assumptions related to

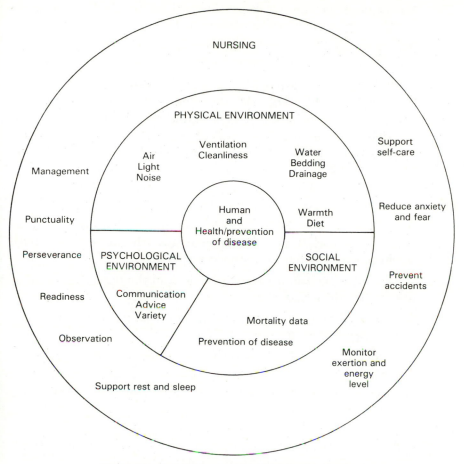

Figure 4-2. Interpretive model of Nightingale's theory.

the concepts identified within the model. She derived these from her experience in caring for the ill and observing the behavior of nurses and physicians. These assumptions need to be viewed in the context of her description of the four major nursing concepts—environment, nursing, health, and humans. The following are some of these assumptions. Note the italicized words which represent the major concept/s within each of these assumptions from Nightingale's *Notes on Nursing.*

In certain diseased states much less *heat* is produced than in health, and there is a constant tendency to the decline and ultimate extinction of the vital powers by the call made upon them to sustain the heat of the body. (p. 17)

You may expect the weak patients will suffer *cold* much more in the morning than in the evening (p 18).

Whatever a patient can do for himself, it is better, i.e. less *anxiety,* for him to do for himself (p 38).

Apprehension, uncertainty, waiting, expectations, fear of surprise, do a patient more harm than any *exertion* (p 38).

Anything which wakes a patient suddenly out of his sleep will invariably put him into a state of greater excitement, do him more serious, aye, and lasting mischief than any continuous *noise,* however loud (p 44).

If a patient is waked after a few hours' instead of a few minutes' *sleep* he is much more likely to sleep again (p 44).

A healthy person who sleeps during the day will lose sleep at night while with a sick person generally, the more they *sleep,* the better they will be able to sleep (p 45).

Variety of form and brillancy of colour in the objects presented to patients are actual means of recovery (p 59).

*Sleep*lessness in the early night is from excitement generally and is increased by tea or coffee (p 77).

The cheerfulness of a room, the usefulness of *light* in treating disease is all important (p 85).

A dirty carpet literally infects the room unless it is taken up two or three times a year to *clean* (p 89).

There is scarcely a greater worry (*fear*) which invalids have to endure than the incurable hopes of friends, visitors, and attendants when they make light of danger and exaggerate the probabilities of recovery (p 96).

In reviewing these assumptions, it is evident that the focus is on nursing's role in relation to the care of the ill. Nursing activities that conserve the patient's energy and reduce anxiety and fear or prevent illness are emphasized. Many of these assumptions appear to be based on common sense and are quite logical. Thus, many respond to them as obvious and believe that they are practical today.

Application to Nursing Process

Although Nightingale did not utilize the term *nursing process,* her approach to sound observations and common sense is very supportive of the process. Most of the data obtained and observations made would be based on the condition of the patient and the physical environment. The nurse's implementation of care would relate to affecting the immediate physical environment and preserving the patient's vital powers so that the reparative process can occur. (See Table 4-1).

This approach to nursing clearly evidences the difference between medicine and nursing, which is probably one of Nightingale's major contributions to the discipline. The nursing process focuses on the patient as a person experiencing a reparative process (disease) and

Table 4-1

Nightingale's Theory

Nursing Process	Focus	Examples
Assessment	Data collected through the observation of the sick:	
	effect of physical environment on reparative process	Does noise level keep patient awake?
		Is there proper ventilation and warmth in the room?
		Does sunlight improve the patient's outlook?
		Are the means to satisfy the patient (such as water) near them so they can meet their own needs?
		Is the environment clean and safe from infection?
	of food and fluids	Is the choice of diet appropriate for the patient in relation to ability to handle food?
		Does the food provide nutrition?
		When does the patient eat best?
		What effect does coffee and tea have on the patient's ability to rest?
	level of anxiety/fear	Do visitors whisper in the presence of the patient?
		Are nurses trustworthy in being punctual and ready to assist the patient when necessary?
		Are communications honest in relationship to the patient's interest in own condition?
		What observations can be made during the daily bath or in talking with the patient that demonstrate the level of anxiety?
	effect of illness on the mind	What effect does fever have on the patient's behavior?
		How does the patient react to pain?

Table 4-1 *(cont.)*

Nursing Process	Focus	Examples
Diagnosis	Needs of patient and level of vital powers as affected by the environment.	Need for warmth, ventilation, sleep, and food. Level of energy available. Reaction to discomfort/pain.
Plan	As based on observations and related to modifications within the environment	Increase the sunlight in the room and reduce the level of noise. Provide patient with energy-saving activities. Place patient in a comfortable position. Decrease/increase use of coffee/tea. Do not awaken during initial periods of sleep.
	communication	Sit and discuss with patient the need for variety to avoid boredom Create a stimulating-healing environment.
Implementation	Modify environment and/or nursing approach	Move a patient to another room. Offer modified diet. Support visitors and family members as they will assist in reducing patient anxiety.
Evaluation	Reassess previous observations for their effect on the patient since changes in the environment have occurred	Is the environment improving the patient's condition and facilitating the reparative process?

not on the disease of an anatomical structure or the physiology of a person as does medicine. Since patients are literally thought to heal themselves for the most part, the role of the nurse in supporting that healing process is a professional one.

In thinking about this approach to nursing, it is interesting to assess the modern hospital of today, especially the intensive care units, in relation to the effects of the environment on the level of anxiety and the recovery of the patient. The question arises: Would Nightingale's theory require us to modify some of the units within a hospital so much as to reshape it dramatically? Admittedly, hospitals are cleaner today than they were in 1860, and they do provide for clean water and proper drainage, yet most hospitals do not allow for fresh air, the reduction of disturbing noises that come from cardiac monitors in intensive care units, or adequate choices of food and eating times. (Do most nurses truly support self-care, monitor noise carefully, monitor sleep-wake patterns, and reduce the patient's fear when they communicate?)

Evaluation

In writing her observations, Nightingale probably would not have identified them as the basis of a nursing theory. Yet she does provide basic concepts and propositions that can be validated and used for practice in nursing. Thus, this is a descriptive theory that provides us with a way of thinking about nursing or a frame of reference that focuses on patients and their environment. This theory is unique to nursing and provides the foundation for later nursing theories. The focus on the human/patient, his state of health, and the role of the nurse permeates all nursing theories that follow. The identification of the difference between medicine and nursing is also a constant.

Concepts

The concepts range from empirical to abstract. The most abstract are *health, anxiety,* and *vital powers.* They are not clearly defined, nor do they have specific characteristics that help one in utilizing them for nursing practice. The concept *health* is one of the most commonly used abstract concepts within the nursing theories; thus, it is hard to distinguish and has different meanings to those reading the theories, leaving confusion in the minds of nurses. The meaning of emotionally charged words such as *anxiety* and *fear* are not offered by Nightingale. Other theorists, especially those oriented toward psychology, do provide clear definitions.

Most of the concepts—such as *ventilation, cleanliness, noise,* and *light*—are inferential, because they can be measured indirectly. The more the concept has characteristics that can be measured, the greater the clarity for nursing practice. Yet, since nursing is a caring profession and highly dependent on an interpersonal communication process, more abstract concepts will emerge. Only through more and better research will these abstract concepts such as *health* be truly useful in practice.

Model

Since Nightingale did not specifically develop a model to demonstrate the relationship between the concepts, an interpretative model may not truly reflect her writings. Admittedly, certain misconceptions could easily evolve within the model developed. For example, ventilation and clean air are stressed over and over again, yet simply reviewing the model would not project such an emphasis.

Also, nursing does relate to the patient directly, especially in the area of observation, but the model does not clearly show such a relationship since the outer circle of *nursing* is not specifically connected to the inner circle of *human*. What is important to realize is that models such as this one assist in finding relationships between the concepts but are not a fine art and have imperfections. Thus, the propositions or assumptions that evolve from a model and that appear logical need to be viewed as tentative conclusions that must be tested in nursing practice as well as researched. They do serve as a foundation for caring for human beings, however, which is essential to nursing practice today.

Propositions

Nightingale's propositions are easy to understand, especially because much of the terminology is familiar to us, and because there are no coined words. The use of a common language within nursing theories facilitates understanding. Words such as *heat, sleep, clean,* and *light* are relatively easy to understand, and most of us would agree on their definitions. However, the degree of heat or light, the amount of sleep needed, and the quality of cleanliness are interpretive, and that is where judgments differ in terms of evaluating the environment and meeting the patient's needs. The propositions are also specific enough to be tested in a nursing situation in a one-to-one relationship with the patient. Although they appear to reflect basic common sense, the obvious is not always clear to us if we are not aware of what observations we need to make. Are nurses usually aware of the impact they have on patients when they awaken them ten minutes after they have fallen into a deep sleep to give them an injection? Do nurses understand the anxiety that patients experience when they are told that everything is fine and that they are improving despite increased long-term pain? Thus, the propositions within the theory are more than just statements offered for one's intellectual consideration. They reflect important assumptions that must be practiced until they are shown to be inaccurate. The results of practicing with this theory should be that the patient will be supported during the reparative process, nature will take its course, and a state of health will follow.

REFERENCES

Nightingale, F., *Notes on Nursing: What It Is and What It Is Not.* New York: Dover Publications, 1969.

5

NEED-ORIENTED THEORIES

INTRODUCTION

The most dominant theme within nursing theories until recently was the concept of *need*. This concept is abstract, so the image created by the use of the term differs. Thus, in order to understand its meaning and make it a useful way of thinking about human beings and their needs, specific criteria or characteristics must be developed. Murray states that *need* is a hypothetical concept, an assumption which he makes from his observations that needs do exist (Murray 1938, p. 60). Maslow believes that humans are motivated by a variety of needs and drives (Maslow 1954). Both of these psychologists provided the foundation for the development of nursing theories for practice.

Historical development validates the fact that the sequence of scientific thinking about human needs is not a new concept (Table 5-1). Many scientists have defined their characteristics with some uniformity and some differences. Thus, in understanding the definition of *needs* as presented by Murray and Maslow, it becomes easier to clarify how nursing theorists incorporate Murray's and Maslow's definitions into their theories so that the concept can be incorporated into the reality of practice.

Table 5-1

Historical Development of Need-Oriented
Nursing Theories

Theory	Theorist and Date	Major Theme
Health-related theories	Murray—1938	Theory of personality
	Maslow—1954	Motivation and personality
Nursing theories	Henderson—1955	Assist patients to meet fourteen identified needs
	Abdellah—1960	List twenty-one nursing problems related to patients' needs
	Orlando—1961	Assist patients who cannot meet their own needs
	Wiedenbach—1964	Humans have a need for help
	Orem—1971	Human beings have self-care needs which are universal, developmental, and related to health deviation
	Kinlein—1977	Self-care practices benefit health state

Criteria

In reviewing Table 5-2, which offers the definitions put forth by the theorists, it is evident that without specific characteristics or criteria for the abstract concept of *need,* there is little clarity. Murray identifies a need as a force or drive; Maslow focuses on motivation, and they both relate the term *behavior* to need. Actually, the dictionary definition is supportive of all the other definitions and provides the criteria upon which to base a discussion of the concept. For example, *needs* are physiological or psychological requirements according to the dictionary, and they are viscerogenic or psychogenic according to Murray. The nursing theorists consistently identify the physical, biological, and socio-psychological needs of humans. The dictionary speaks to needs as conditions requiring supply or relief. Orlando and Wiedenbach relate needs to requirements that if met relieve distress or create comfort. Again, the concept remains abstract in its meaning and requires greater clarity through the identification of characteristics.

Incorporated into the meaning of *need* are the four basic concepts of nursing. *Humans* are described as having needs, *health* is viewed as having one's needs met to maintain life, *nursing* has the responsibility to meet human needs, and the *environment* affects humans' ability to meet their needs. Thus, the concept of need is very appropriate as a framework for nursing.

This chapter will examine eight need-oriented theories. Two, those of Murray and Maslow, are basically psychological theories, al-

Table 5-2

Definition of the Concept *Need*

Source	Definition
Dictionary—common language usage	Lack of something requisite, desirable, or useful. Physiological or psychological requirement for the well-being of an organism. Condition requiring supply or relief.
Murray	A hypothetical force (a drive, need, or propensity) within an organism that affects behavior. These behaviors are either viscerogenic, arising from within the body, or psychogenic, arising from the mind, involving the initiation and cessation of activity.
Maslow	Humans have needs, desires, or drives that are basically hierarchical that motivate their behaviors.
Henderson	Humans basically perform fourteen activities which reflect their needs.
Abdellah	Patients have physical, biological, and social-psychological needs.
Orlando	A requirement of the patient which, if supplied, relieves or diminishes his immediate distress or improve his immediate sense of adequacy or well-being.
Wiedenbach	Anything the individual requires to maintain or sustain himself comfortably or capably in his situation.
Orem	Human beings have common needs for the intake of materials and for bringing about and maintaining living conditions that support the health process.
Kinlein	Utilizes Orem's definition and focuses on client's ability to recognize and communicate their needs.

though they have implications for health. The theories of Henderson, Abdellah, Orlando, Wiedenbach, Orem, and Kinlein are nursing theories. Analysis of each theory will include four aspects: a description, including identifying major concepts; one or more models; application to nursing process; and evaluation.

HENRY MURRAY: DESCRIPTION
OF THE THEORY AND APPLICATION
TO THE NURSING PROCESS

Murray, a medical psychologist, was influenced by Carl Jung and his writings on psychotherapy. In his text *Explorations in Personality,* which will be quoted frequently, he offers general propositions (assumptions) which he views as provisional and basic to his definition and description of the characteristics of needs. The following are some of his most significant ideas related to nursing theories:

> An organism is whole and the parts are mutually related. An understanding of the whole being is as essential to understanding the parts as the parts are to understanding the whole.

Basic to all need-oriented nursing theories is the assumption that we provide nursing care to individuals in terms of their specific needs (the parts) while viewing the individual as a whole organism.

> An organism has from the beginning rhythms of activity and rest.

As will be noted later, especially in relation to nursing theories, the need for mobility in the form of exercise, sleep, and rest is a consistent theme.

> An organism is within a changing environment which largely determines its behavior.

Nursing theories utilizing the need concept, except Kinlein's, generally focus on nursing care within the hospital environment, which is a major change for the patient. Thus, behaviors in relation to need should be viewed from the perspective of the individual's reaction to that environment. Basically, need theorists in nursing do not emphasize the environment as providing the focal point for attention in the care of clients.

> The stimulus situation is that part of the total environment to which humans attend and react.

The stimulus could be viewed as an unmet need, as discussed, for example, by Orem and Henderson. For Abdellah, this stimulus or unmet need creates a nursing problem.

> The existence of an organism depends on its adaptive response in order to restore equilibrium, avoid injury or attain objects that are of benefit to development.

Basic to Murray's needs classification are psychological and safety needs, which focus on balance/equilibrium within the individual. The physiological needs identified by Henderson and Abdellah, such as the need for air and fluid, also reflect an emphasis on internal equilibrium.

In summary, the propositions identified by Murray focus on the human as a whole related to its parts, having rhythms, experiencing environmental stimuli, and responding in an adaptive manner to a changing environment. The major concepts seem to be *whole, rhythm, stimuli, change,* and *environment.*

Model

Some concepts, especially those that are abstract, such as *need,* require clarification through the use of concepts interrelated through a model. It would be helpful to view a model that supports Murray's propositions. For example, the linear and directional model shown in Figure 5-1 supports Murray's focus.

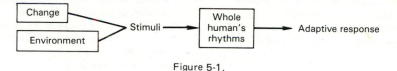

Figure 5-1.

The concepts within the model assist in clarifying the human's response to stimuli, but deriving the meaning of the specific concepts is almost an endless task. Can you answer the following questions? Does change involve simply a normal developmental process and growth, or a crisis, or both? Is the environment within the understanding of the human being, or is it universal? How is the adaptive response related to physiology and culture? Answers to all of these are uncertain. Basically, Murray's propositions attempt to explain the behavior of humans so that we can understand their needs.

Needs Categories

Murray divides needs into two major categories, viscerogenic and psychogenic (see Table 5-3). As a needs classification system, it provides a view of Murray's perception of the total needs of humans. It contains one of the most extensive lists of mental and emotional needs. The major subcategories under *viscerogenic* reflect intake, output, and harm. It is not clear why harm, which speaks to the avoidance of pain, physical injury, illness, or death is more related to physical needs than environmental ones.

Table 5-3

Needs Categories

Viscerogenic (physical)	Psychogenic (mental/emotional)
Lacks (leading to intakes)	Inanimate object associations
Inspiration (oxygen)	Acquisition (gain property)
Water	Conservance (preserve property)
Food	Order (clean, precise)
Sentience (sensual gratification such as	Retention (hoard property)
taste/touch)	Construction (organize, build)
Distensions (leading to outputs)	Ambition
Secretion (life sources)	Superiority (ambitious attitude)
Sex	Achievement (power over things, people,
Lactation	objects)
Expiration (CO_2)	Recognition (demand respect, seek
Excretion (waste)	praise)
Urination	Exhibition (shock others, attract
Defecation	attention)
Harms (leading to retractions)	Defense of status/avoid humiliation
Noxavoidance (avoid noxious stimuli)	Inviolacy (prevent loss of self-respect)
Heatavoidance (avoid heat)	Infavoidance (avoid failure, shame)
Coldavoidance (avoid cold)	Defendance (avoid blame, make excuses)
Harmavoidance (avoid physical pain)	Counteraction (select hardest tasks,
	retaliating)
	Human power exertion
	Dominance (influence, lead others)
	Deference (cooperate with leader)
	Similance (empathize, emulate)
	Autonomy (resist influence, coercion)
	Contrarience (unconventional views)
	Sado-masochistic
	Aggression (punish)
	Abasement (comply, self-deprecation)
	Blamavoidance (well-behaved)
	Affection between people
	Affiliation (form friendships)
	Rejection (ignore, exclude)
	Nurturance (protect helpless)
	Succorance (be dependent)
	Play (seek amusement, relax)
	Social life
	Cognizance (inquiring, curious)
	Exposition (demonstrate, relate facts)

The seven subcategories under *psychogenic* are basically behavioral, with no positive or negative value placed on them. These subcategories are further defined; for example, *ambition* includes superiority, achievement, recognition, and exhibition.

Evaluation

Whenever we have a classification system based on needs, we must ask whether it is an all-inclusive list or whether there are needs that are not mentioned. If the list is complete, we can utilize this classification system whenever we relate to or observe other human beings in order to identify which need is affecting their behavior. Also, since most of the concepts or words used to explain the categories and subcategories are more abstract than empirical, especially within the emotional area, there is a tendency to place more specific newly identified needs in a particular category, with the new needs assuming the meaning of the category. Murray, within his text, identifies more specifics and explains the meanings of such words as *achievement,* which includes such things as the kinds of achievements (such as athletic success), the kinds of traits (such as ambition), and the kinds of actions (such as intense, prolonged, and repeated efforts to accomplish something difficult). There is also the problem of determining whether some needs fit under one category or under several. For example, sex is viewed as a distension and as physically oriented, but how does that need relate to human power and affection? Murray does acknowledge an interrelationship and fusion among needs. (Fusion occurs when a single action satisfies two or more needs at the same time.) He speaks of some needs as having a definite and sometimes enduring relationship, as well as of needs coming in conflict with one another, creating misery and neurosis.

ABRAHAM MASLOW: DESCRIPTION OF THE THEORY

The focus of Maslow's text, *Motivation and Personality,* is on the fully human person taking a step away from the limitations of behaviorism and Freudianism. Maslow, like Murray, provides some important assumptions/propositions about motivation that help to explain the basis of his approach to human needs. You will note the similarity to the propositions offered by Murray some sixteen years before.

"The individual is an integrated, organized whole." This proposition is frequently stated, but often ignored. The whole individual, not the parts of the individual, is seen as being motivated. The example offered in Maslow's text relates to a person's being hungry and its impact on the person's stomach, but we must also recognize that hunger affects the individual's perceptions, memory, and thinking capacity. In other words, a person is hungry all over. The typical drive or desire is most often the need of the whole person.

"The average desires that we have in our daily lives are usually a means to an end, rather than the end itself." This supports the idea that we cannot superficially identify a specific need, meet it, and assume that we understand the person's goal or the other needs behind it. Thus, the study of motivation in relation to needs is essential and relates to some understanding of the conscious life of the individual.

"Fundamental or ultimate desires of all human beings do not differ significantly due to our cultural influences." The idea here is that human beings, especially those within the same culture, are much more alike than one would think at first. This validates categorizing needs that are reflective of us all, but we should be careful to recognize that any approach to classifying needs is basically cultural.

"Acts or a conscious wish usually have multiple motivations." In order to more totally understand needs and desires, it is important to recognize the many ways in which a particular act may be influenced by multiple motivations. Sexual desires may be influenced by our motivation for closeness, friendliness, safety, love, or any combination of these. Humans are too complex in their behavior for a single motivation to lead to a single need and act.

"Motivation is a constant, never ending, fluctuating and complex organismic state of affairs." Thus, since our motivations are dynamic, our meeting of human needs is continuous and requires modification and increasing clarity in relation to any individual. There is no static state of human need gratification. Time does not stand still.

"Human beings are never satisfied except in a relative or one-step-along-the-path fashion." Satisfaction of a need can only occur for a short time before another need takes place. Need satisfaction is a continuous process that involves arranging a sort of hierarchy in which one need is given precedence over the other.

"Drives arrange themselves in a hierarchy of specificity and should not be listed." Maslow seems to differ from Murray in his thinking about creating a list of needs, for several reasons. First, a list implies equality of various drives. Second, it implies that one need can be isolated from another, which neglects to adequately take into account the dynamic nature of drives. Thus, since drives in and of themselves are constantly shifting in priority and are inseparable, specific lists are not appropriate to Maslow. He believes that we can classify life's motivations, influenced by goals or needs. Thus, the discussion tries to separate drives and needs as different, because according to Maslow we can list needs, not drives. Again the lack of clarity of the terms *needs* versus *drives* leaves one confused. Maslow believes that we could come up with one to one million drives depending on the specificity of the analysis. Thus his presentation, which is to be discussed next, offers a series of prioritized needs that are more limited than Murray's.

"Within the environment, the need not only organizes its action efficiently with great variation, but it also organizes and even creates the external reality." Emphasis is placed on human motivation within the context of the organism's partly creating barriers or identifying its objects of value. Thus, the environment's impact is minimized and the focus on the individual is maximized. Maslow would state that there is too much emphasis on and preoccupation with the exterior. Surely, he would disagree with Nightingale's strong emphasis on the environment.

"The organism is most unified when it experiences success, joy or is creative, or when a major problem, threat or emergency exists." Humans can act in a nonunified way in their daily lives and in their habits, and when they are weak or helpless, yet when in a healthy state, they will appear more integrated and whole. This is significant because Maslow's primary assumption recognizes humans as integrated and organized, while this assumption offers clarity as to when he perceives the organism is capable of projecting that wholeness.

In summary, Maslow's propositions focus on the similarities of the unified organism/human who is constantly motivated to meet changing needs. Note that the emphasis is not on the environment, nor is there a belief that a long list of drives is helpful; this gives clues to the meaning of needs. For example, both boredom and interest are observable and relate to multiple needs.

Models

In developing a model to express the major concepts provided by Maslow, emphasis is on the characteristics of humans rather than on explaining specific needs. Simply stated, humans have the motivation to meet changing needs, as shown in Figure 5-2.

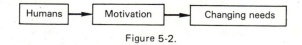

Figure 5-2.

Table 5-4 identifies the five major needs put forth by Maslow. The examples listed do not attempt to offer a total picture of all the

Table 5-4

Maslow's Needs and Related Concepts

Need	Related Concepts	Characteristics
Physiological	Hunger/food Sex Thirst/fluid Activity Stimulation	Some physiological needs are universal since they can be isolated and localized somatically, e.g., hunger and thirst. They are the most consistent of all needs. Gratification of these needs releases the organism to focus on higher needs, such as those related to social goals.
Safety	Security Stability Dependency Protection Freedom from fear, anxiety, chaos Need for structure, order, law, limits Strength in protection	Safety has basically the same characteristics as physiological needs. Safety needs can be exclusive organizers of behaviors, creating a view of the total organism as safety seeking. They can be strong determinants of the human's view of the world and its future. There is a preference for the familiar and known which provides meaning.
Belongingness and love	Affection Place in group or family Avoid pain of loneliness, rejection, friendlessness Intimacy	When physiological and safety needs are met, these needs emerge with intensity. Love is not synonomous with sex. Love needs involve both giving and receiving. Humans who have led loving lives and have loved and been loved need love *less* because they already have enough.
Esteem (self-respect)	Desire for strength, achievement, adequacy, mastery and competence, independence and freedom Desire for reputation or prestige status, fame and glory, dominance, recognition, attention, importance, dignity, or appreciation	Thwarting these needs produces feelings of inferiority, weakness, and helplessness. Competence and achievement that are based on will power, determination, and responsibility come from one's real self and offer deserved respect from others.

Table 5-4 (cont.)

Need	Related Concepts	Characteristics
Self-actualization	Doing what one is fitted for and being true to one's own nature Involves self-fulfillment Becoming everything that one is capable of becoming	Individual differences are greatest at this level. This need emerges when there is real satisfaction of the other needs

possible needs under the major need, but only to help clarify its meaning. The characteristics of each of the major needs support the assumptions previously made, especially in relationship to the emergence of a hierarchical structure of needs. Maslow repeatedly states that it is only when the lower needs, such as physiological needs, are met that the higher needs, such as those for self-actualization, can be met. A foundational model that reflects this approach is shown in Figure 5-3. This model provides a view of each concept and indicates that physiological needs are basic to safety needs; physiological and safety needs to needs for love; and so on. Self-actualization is at the top because it is viewed as the highest of all needs.

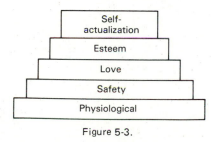

Figure 5-3.

Maslow is quick to recognize that although his hierarchical order of the five needs applies to most people, there are exceptions. At times, for example, self-esteem appears more important than love. Such a prioritization is evident when a husband spends most of his waking hours on the job in order to achieve status and prestige and appears to ignore his loved ones. Intensely creative people or people who have had their lower needs met will forego some basic needs for their ideals which reflect their strong values. Table 5-4 identifies Maslow's list of needs, those specific concepts related to each need, and the characteristics of those concepts. This represents the analysis of his major concepts so that the concepts can be better understood.

Table 5-5

Maslow's Theory—The Conceptual Difference

Need	Physiological	Safety	Love	Self-Esteem	Self-Actualization
Type of concept	Empirical—easier to define and observe	Inferential—indirectly observable			Abstract—most difficult to define and observe
Degree of satisfaction	Greatest potential satisfaction level (85%)	(70%)	(50%)	(40%)	Least potential satisfaction level (10%)
Degree of variance between cultures	Most universal in nature	← →			Least universal in nature
Level of consciousness	Individuals function by habit and are in least conscious state, unless there is a problem	← →			Individuals most conscious of the need
Environmental influence	Require less externally positive conditions, such as a satisfactory political or educational state, for the individual to meet the need	← →			Require best environmental conditions for achievement of this need

Human development	Basic to human evolutionary development and similar to other living things Orientation is greater at birth	⟷	Characteristic only of human development and usually increases its potential for achievement with in-creasing age
Reaction to unmet needs	Most imperative that needs be met Most urgent and objective	⟷	Deprivation of need does not produce an emergency reaction Less urgent and more subjective
Relationship to health	Most essential to a healthy state and can support the meeting of higher need	⟷	Living at a higher need level means greater biological efficiency, longevity, less disease, and so on.
Ability to identify	More localized, more tan-gible and limited in scope	⟷	More generalized, broad, and unlimited in scope

An individual who starves to death for a great social cause is very willing to give up both the physiological and safety needs.

In viewing Maslow's needs, it is helpful to understand the conceptual differences among each of the needs (Table 5-5). Although viewing these needs on a continuum is simplistic, which often leads to some misinterpretation, it is an effective way of trying to understand which needs provide greater clarity for practice. As with most concepts (as discussed in Chapter 2), those that are empirical and mean similar things to most of us are easier to use and understand. This is evident in terms of the degree to which a particular need must be satisfied before one can move to meet a higher-level need. For example, Maslow stipulates that if eighty-five percent of our physiological needs are met and seventy percent of our safety needs are met, we can focus on our love needs. It is interesting to note that he recognizes the limited degree of potential forces to self-actualize. Maybe this is the highest of all human goals.

In reviewing Table 5-5, the following should be evident to the reader. Those needs (physiological) which are mostly empirical tend to be easier to satisfy, most universal, limited, dealt with mostly through habit, less reactive to external forces, and more instinctive and essential for health, while the most abstract need (self-actualization) has characteristics that are basically the opposite of those of the empirical needs.

Love needs can be assessed by inferential behaviors; its concepts fall somewhere between empirical and abstract. Thus love as a need has a more limited potential for achievement than food but a greater potential for achievement than self-fulfillment. In other words, it is easier to meet the need for food than the need for self-actualization.

> Needs have an effect on and are affected by the degree of satisfaction reaction to the state of other needs, the environment/culture, state of health, state of consciousness and the level of the individual's growth and development.

Maslow believes that although one should not identify the many specific drives/needs, certain behaviors should and can be observed when there is basic need gratification. For example, feelings of physical contentment follow when the need for food is satisfied, and feelings of security and peace occur when the safety needs are met. Individuals who are more demonstrative, friendly, loving, creative, and relaxed obviously have had enough of their needs met. When individuals appear to have a general feeling of well-being and project that image, we usually recognize that the level of need satisfaction is high.

Evalution

In comparing Murray to Maslow, it is evident that many basic ideas are similar, including the following:

—Understanding of humans' changing drives/needs.

—Focusing on the whole human being, but categorizing needs for a physical, psychological, and sociological framework.

—Attempting to bring clarity to the abstract concept of need by identifying specific needs and/or categories of needs.

Their differences relate to whether we should offer a detailed list of needs, as Murray suggests, or prioritize categories of needs, as Maslow recommends, in order to understand the human personality. Both use abstract concepts, but Murray offers more specific criteria for understanding their meaning. Both focus primarily on physiologi-cal needs—Murray on the need for air, food, water, Maslow on the basic needs for food, fluid, and activity. Secondary are Murray's no-tion of harm and Maslow's ideas about safety. Admittedly, Murray has not actually prioritized these needs, but he presents them first in his writings. Murray relates to ambition and achievement, Maslow to self-esteem; Murray to affiliation for affection, Maslow to love and belonging.

Application to Nursing Process

The approach used by all the nursing theorists who are need-oriented is very similar to the idea presented by Murray and Maslow. The major ideas about nursing and the emphasis of these theories have already been presented in Chapter 1. It is now helpful to iden-tify and compare their differences. From a general model approach we can easily visualize some of the similarities and differences within approaches to needs. At times, the terminology may differ more than the ideas presented. (See Table 5-6.) These models shown in Table 5-6 validate that all the theorists focus on human needs. In terms of the nurse's role, all—except Kinlein, the most recent need theorist, and probably Henderson—give the major responsibility to the nurse to identify the individual's need rather than share the re-sponsibilities with the patient/client. While Henderson and Orem identify specific needs and Abdellah specifies problems that could be translated into specific needs, as Murray did, other theorists such as Orlando and Wiedenbach make little attempt to develop lists of

Table 5-6

Modeling Nursing Theories Related to Need

Theorist	Model	Focus
Henderson	Human needs help ⟷ Nurse provides help 14 Patient needs	Humans and nurse interact to provide for the 14 patient needs.
Abdellah	Nurse → 21 Nursing problems → Provides total health needs	The nurse, through the use of a 21-nursing-problems approach, provides for the total health needs of the patient.
Orlando	Nurse → Relieves immediate distress → Improves sense of well-being	The nurse relieves immediate stress to improve sense of well-being.
Wiedenbach	Individual behavioral stimuli → Need for help → Nurse meets need	The individual demonstrates through a behavioral stimulus the need for help, and the nurse meets that need.
Orem	Nurse → Individual need for self-care → Universal need / Health deviation / Self-care need / Developmental self-care needs → Overcome self-care deficits	The nurse identifies the individual need for self-care in the framework of universal health deviation and developmental self-care needs in order to overcome the patient's self-care deficits.
Kinlein	Identification of client self-care need by nurse with client → Assess client's assets and deficits → Nurse assists client toward health	The nurse and the client identify and assess client's self-care needs to achieve health.

needs, similar to Maslow's approach. All the models give the nurse a sense of direction or a goal, which is either to simply provide for the needs (Orlando) or to focus on getting clients/patients to learn through self-care or to provide for their own needs (Orem and Kinlein).

In utilizing any of these models and theories, certain assumptions/propositions have been made. For example, all humans have needs and want those needs met. The nurse has the primary goal of focusing on identifying/assessing human needs. One should also recognize that certain broad concepts, such as the environment, are not stressed. The need approach does not provide much clarity in terms of health and its meaning. Of the four concepts basic to nursing practice (health, nursing, human, and environment), nursing and human are central to need theories; health is given minimal emphasis, and there is little real mention of the environment. As a result, the use of this theoretical approach will probably sometimes lead to inadequate processing of information. The most appropriate theoretical approaches would give some emphasis to all four nursing concepts.

VIRGINIA HENDERSON: DESCRIPTION OF THE THEORY

Henderson, in her *Textbook of the Principles and Practice of Nursing* (written with Harmer), offers a specific definition of nursing, in which she analyzes the unique function of nursing.

> To assist the individual, sick or well, in the performance of those activities contributing to health or its recovery (or to a peaceful death) that he would perform unaided if he had the necessary strength, will, or knowledge. It is likewise her function to help the individual gain independence as rapidly as possible. (p. 4)

The major concepts that relate to this theory as seen within the definition of nursing are *individual,* described as sick or well; *nurse,* as an assisting person who performs activities; *health,* as the ability of the individual to function unaided with the necessary strength, knowledge, and will; and *independence* as a goal. The most empirical concept is the term *nurse.* For Henderson *nurse* means the person who serves as a substitute for what the patient lacks. By inference we can gather that a person dressed in white within a hospital or in a blue uniform within a community health agency who cares for the sick or well is a nurse. When Henderson's book was written in 1955, the vast majority of nurses worked in hospitals and were easy to identify. Nevertheless, many workers wear white—laboratory technicians, hairdressers, and nutritionists, for example. Therefore our mental image of a nurse also needs to include someone (nurse) in relation to a sick or well individual. The concept *nurse* cannot stand without the other concepts in the definition.

The most abstract or poorly developed concept is *health*. "The individual's ability to function" is basically inadequate as the criterion/characteristic for the term *health*. Also, the individual's perception of his ability to function and the nurse's perception may differ substantially. As a result it would be difficult to distinguish whether an individual had a state of health, since we do not know what Henderson really meant. Individuals who are confined to wheelchairs and are totally rehabilitated but require some assistance may be viewed as unhealthy, while those who are completely able to physically function may be emotionally disturbed but perceived as healthy. Basically, if one focuses on physiological health and on caring for basic needs as described by Murray and Maslow, the term *health* becomes clearer. The concept *individual* (human) is characterized as one who is either sick or well and has a state of independence. The word *well* probably is related to the word *health*.

The nurse is the focus of the theory. Henderson's motive in presenting her ideas was to clarify the role of the nurse rather than fully explain the characteristics of the individual or health.

Models

In relating the four basic concepts in nursing theory to Henderson's specific definition, the following linear and directional model (Fig. 5-4) could be used:

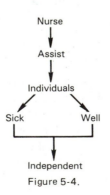

Figure 5-4.

From this model certain assumptions/propositions can be developed.

Nursing can assist individuals.

Individuals are in a state of sickness or wellness.

Sick or well individuals can become independent.

Although the concepts related to health, sickness, and wellness are relatively abstract and thus unclear, these propositions are readily verifiable and are generally accepted as truths. Nurses do help individuals, especially those who are sick, become more independent by encouraging them to care for themselves. Thus as a theory, at least through its definition, it does describe nursing.

Another model has been developed by the Nursing Development Conference Group. As shown in Figure 5-5, it is also linear and directional.

This model gives a pictorial view of the definition and the rela-

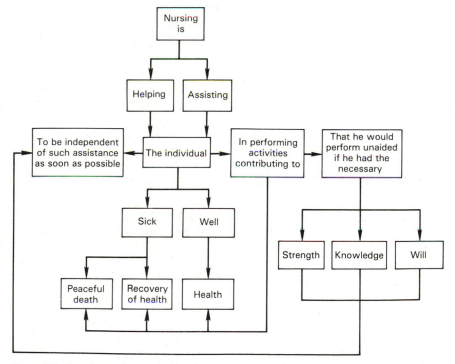

Figure 5-5. Dominant themes in Henderson's concept of nursing; formalization of patient agency theme and subsumption of health themes. From Nursing Development Conference Group—*Concept Formalization in Nursing Process and Product,* p. 56, Little, Brown, & Co., 1973.

tionship between the concepts/words within it. The arrows give a sense of direction leading the nurse to the goal of the individual's independence. Note that the propositions within this model are multiple. Review the model by following the arrows.

Nursing is helping and assisting the individual.

The individual is affected by the nurse, the performance of activities, and a sense of independence.

Individuals are sick and well.

Individuals who are sick will experience either a recovery of health or a peaceful death.

Individuals have the necessary strength, knowledge, and will to be independent.

Again the latter model reemphasizes Henderson's theoretical approach, which is to explain the function of nursing.

Henderson does specify the activities or conditions that require nursing assistance. These are usually spoken of as Henderson's fourteen needs; they are listed in Henderson's *The Nature of Nursing.*

1. Breathe normally.
2. Eat and drink adequately.
3. Eliminate body wastes.
4. Move and maintain desirable posture.
5. Sleep and rest.
6. Select suitable clothing.
7. Maintain body temperature.
8. Keep body clean and well groomed and protect the integument.
9. Avoid environmental dangers and avoid injuring others.
10. Communicate with others in expressing emotions, needs, fears or opinions.
11. Worship according to faith.
12. Work at something providing a sense of accomplishment.
13. Play or participate in various forms of recreation.
14. Learn, discover, or satisfy curiosity that leads to normal development and health and use of the available health facilities.

These activities/conditions, which are basically needs, relate very closely to Maslow's in that they evidence a hierarchical need approach. Physiological needs are Henderson's 1 through 7, safety needs are 8 and 9, love needs are 10 and 11, the need for esteem is 10, and self-actualization needs are 11 through 14. Henderson does not specifically state that her needs are hierarchical, yet when compared with Maslow's listing, it appears that they are.

Application to Nursing Process

It is not too difficult to use Henderson's theory within the context of the nursing process. Table 5-7 gives some examples of how the theory could be applied to the nursing process. It represents no particular situation, but reflects the emphasis that could be placed on each of the fourteen needs. It is quite possible that an individual could have a poor intake of food, be dehydrated, have difficulty breathing, have a high temperature, and be bored all at the same time. Each need would be handled separately. The relationship between the fourteen needs, aside from their being separated by physiological, social, and emotional need categories, is not clear. For example, what is the relationship between communicating with others and working or worshipping, between being well groomed and selecting suitable clothes? Do poor eating habits lead to poor elimination of wastes?

The following case history may offer some understanding about the use of the theory in a more integrated manner.

Situation: Mr. Rodriguez is admitted to the hospital complaining of pain in the chest and difficulty breathing after a car accident. The physician, after reviewing a series of X rays, makes the diagnosis of fracture of the ribs. The nurse who enters Mr. Rodriguez's room finds him very uncomfortable, lying in a flat position in bed, unable to reach for water, and requesting a urinal. The *initial* focus on the part of the nurse would be as follows:

Assessment—unable to reach water, uncomfortable in a flat position; needs to eliminate urine; breathing is difficult and painful.

Diagnosis—pain on inspiration.

Implementation—raise head of bed until comfortable; place urinal and pitcher of water within easy reach.

Evaluation—reassess ability to breathe easily and achieve some mobility.

Table 5-7

Incorporation of Henderson's Needs
and the Nursing Process

Need	Assessment Data	Nursing Diagnosis	Plan	Implementation	Evaluation
Breathe normally	Note rate, depth, and pattern of breathing	Difficulty breathing Shallow respirations	Identify ways of facilitating breathing	Place individual in a sitting position to facilitate respirations	Reassess ability to breathe normally
Eat and drink adequately	Review daily intake of food and fluid	Dehydration Overweight	Facilitate intake of proper food	Assist the individual in learning to feed self	Reassess whether patient is eating properly
Eliminate body waste	Measure urinary output	Inability to urinate postsurgery	Encourage independent activities that facilitate urination	Assist patient to the bathroom and provide privacy	Continue to measure urinary output
Move and maintain posture	Note posture and ability to ambulate	Difficulty walking Slides down in bed	Support patient when getting in and out of bed	Assist in walking around the immediate environment	Observe for independent activities related to movement
Sleep/rest	Review sleep habits	Insomnia	Provide positive environment	Reassure patient that he will not be disturbed during rest periods	Reassess sleep and rest patterns
Clothing	Check for comfort of bedclothing	Feeling of too much warmth	Provide appropriate bedclothing	Remove blankets and provide a nightshirt	Check to see whether individual is more comfortable
Body temperature	Take temperature	High temperature, sweating, headache	Monitor temperature and fluid intake	Take temperature every four hours Encourage fluids	Reassess if temperature does not return to normal
Cleanliness	Check for body cleanliness and bed sores (decubitus)	Decubitus ulcers on heels; unclean hair causing discomfort	Avoid pressure on heels; provide environment for patient to wash hair	Wash hair; turn individual frequently	Monitor ulcers on heels Observe for increased independence in maintaining cleanliness

Environmental dangers	Check floor for danger of slippery areas	Environment unsafe for walking	Provide safe walking area	Remove water spots from floor	Assess whether individual is aware of environmental hazards
Communicate	Note interaction pattern with family and health care personnel	Unable to communicate with wife concerning state of health	Help patient to identify why he is fearful of talking to his wife about his condition	Sit down in a quiet environment and discuss the individual's feelings and needs	Reassess interaction patterns
Worship	Gather information about patient's feelings about having an abortion	Conflict over religious values regarding abortion	Assist patient to seek religious and other counseling	Provide an appropriate environment to facilitate communication between the patient and the clergy member	Reassess the level of acceptance or nonacceptance of the abortion
Sense of accomplishment	Identify impact of surgery on individual's work	Inability to perform present work and physical labor	Provide a vocational counselor	Schedule a visit with a vocational counselor prior to the individual's returning home	Reassess whether the individual follows up on the visit
Recreation	Observe for feelings of boredom	Inactivity and infrequent interaction with others	Provide opportunities for participation in recreation	Have someone invite patient to participate in social affairs	Reassess effect of increased activity and ability to function independently
Normal development and health	Identify individual's understanding of his illness and of the available resources	Lacks information regarding his condition and the available resources	Plan a learning program	Teach the patient about the impact his illness will have on his activities	Reassess the information learned and needed for health and independence

After the initial assessment, which actually incorporated the first four needs, the nurse would continue to assess Mr. Rodriguez in terms of his ability to communicate, sleep, and so on. Constant reassessment is performed with every interaction, affecting the other stages of the nursing process. For example, new assessment data about his ability to rest will affect the plan and implementation of care. It should be noted that needs are integrated, and one that is unmet has a strong impact on the others. Utilizing each of Henderson's needs in isolation is truly impractical and would lead to inadequate nursing care.

Evaluation

The major concepts of nurse, individual, health, and independence are more abstract than empirical. It is not entirely clear how each relates to the fourteen needs. Among the needs that are either directly measurable (empirical) or indirectly measurable (inferential) are breathing, eating-drinking-eliminating, moving, sleeping, temperature, cleanliness, and changes (1-9). Those that are more abstract are communication, faith, sense of accomplishment, recreation, and curiosity. The latter items are hard to define, and their characteristics differ from individual to individual.

The needs are characteristics of individuals and direct the activities of the nurse. The theory is described with economy of words, and it is rather easy to understand. There is also an unstated hierarchical order to the needs, so although one could infer that Henderson felt that normal breathing was primary while learning was least important, this is probably too simplistic an approach; it may be that some are hierarchical and others are not.

Henderson did not develop models; the models shown in Figures 5-4 and 5-5 represent the writer's interpretation of what Henderson identified as the purpose of nursing. These models lead to some inherent, unusually creative propositions that are verifiable and congruent with existing theories, especially Maslow's. As a theory, it offers a description of events surrounding an individual, especially one who is ill, and explains human beings in terms of needs. This approach assists nursing by giving it a focus that is not disease oriented but more humanistic. For example, instead of emphasizing the diagnosis of pneumonia in the care of the patient, Henderson, like Nightingale, would have the nurse deal with the *patient* as the focus of care by helping him to breathe, eat, and maintain fluid balance, as well as by creating a positive environment.

FAYE G. ABDELLAH:
DESCRIPTION OF THE THEORY

Abdellah, in her book *Patient-Centered Approach to Nursing*, defines nursing as a service to individuals and families, and therefore to society (p. 24). The service is recognized as involving the following:

The recognition of nursing problems as patient problems.

It should be noted that the problems are more nursing's than the patient's. Here the emphasis is on the nurse rather than on the patient.

The decision as to which courses of action to take related to nursing principles.

Again the decision about implementation is the nurse's rather than the patient's.

Offering continuous care of the individual's total health needs.

The emphasis here is on the nurse's providing ongoing care for not only illness needs but all-inclusive health needs.

Providing care continually to relieve pain and discomfort and provide for security.

The relief of pain and discomfort is viewed as one of the major responsibilities of the nurse.

Providing a nursing care plan to meet the patient's individual needs.

This sentence supports the idea that Abdellah is actually need oriented, although she speaks more of problems. The use of these terms without clear definitions leads to confusion. For our purposes and interpretation, *problems* are really nursing problems, and *needs* are basically physical, biological, and social-psychological. The two are very related in Abdellah's theory, as you will note.

Helping the individual to become more self-directing in order to maintain health of mind and body.

This builds on Henderson's orientation toward assisting individuals to become independent so as to achieve the goal of health.

Instructing others to help the individual do for himself what he can within his limits.

This service reinforces the previous statement, integrating self-direction with teaching others to encourage self-help.

Helping individuals adjust to their limitations and emotional problems.

The focus here is on the adjustment to limitations. It is unclear, though, how limitations are either the same as or different from emotional problems.

Working with allied health professions on a local, state, national, and international level to plan for optimum health.

The emphasis here is on groups, rather than individuals, working together to achieve health.

Continuous evaluation and research to improve nursing techniques and develop new techniques to meet health needs of people.

Here Abdellah focuses on universal needs and the technology needed to meet these needs. This service builds on the previous one.

Abdellah also identifies five basic elements needed to provide the service.

1. Mastery of *human skills and relations*—This is particularly true of services such as instructing individuals and families and relating to other health care professionals.
2. *Observation* and *reporting*—Effective communication skills are needed in order to clearly present the signs and symptoms identified.
3. *Interpretation* of *signs* and *symptoms*—The deviations from health and constituent nursing problems require that the nurse observe signs and symptoms in order to identify possible solutions.
4. *Analysis* of nursing problems—This will assist the nurse in selecting a course of action.
5. *Organization*—To ensure a desired outcome.

Effective care takes place when the nurse is able to help the patient return to health.

Models

Incorporated into the nurse's service and the basic elements of that service are a few basic interrelated concepts. The following models are all possible from Abdellah's theory.

A *nondirectional model* would integrate services and then basic elements as shown in Figure 5-6.

This model is *nondirectional* for the most part, although one can assume that health is the end result of self-direction and adjustment. Here, as with Henderson's theory, the concept of health is not well defined. Propositions would speak to a nonlinear relationship between *problem* and *need*—for example, the nonpositional statement that patient care involves nursing problems and patient needs with an emphasis on self-direction and adjustment in order to achieve health.

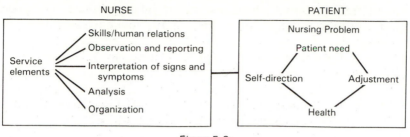

Figure 5-6.

A *linear* model would make a propositional statement that a lack of a patient's meeting those needs leads to a question about the patient's ability for self-direction and adjustment, resulting in change of health as viewed by the nurse through the identification of a nursing problem. The *linear model* shown in Figure 5-7a integrates service (does not include basic elements). *A circular model,* such as Figure 5-7b, shows integration of services.

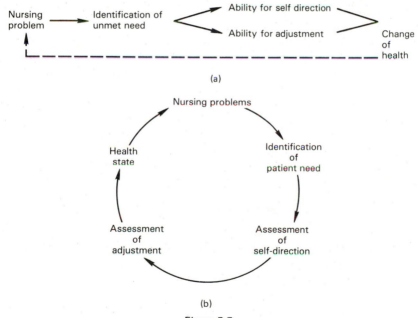

Figure 5-7.

The circular model generally would start with the nursing problem, which assists the nurse to identify a patient need that is not being met. This would lead the nurse (probably through the use of the five basic elements) to assess the patient's self-direction and adjustment ability so that a health state can be determined. The process would continue indefinitely as long as the nurse-patient interaction continued.

The following assumptions/propositions can be drawn from the circular model:

> Nursing problems relate to the needs of the patient in relation to the patient's ability to self-direct and adjust.

> The health state of a patient is influenced by his adjustment and sense of self-direction based on his needs.

There is not a lot of difference between the linear and circular models, except that in the circular model the health state leads to the recognition of a nursing problem, while in the linear model there is a sense of termination in the activity. If a direction line were drawn back to the nursing problem in the linear model (note the dashed line), it would be similar to the circular model, except that unmet need would lead to either assessment or lack of self-direction or adjustment, whereas in the circular model, assessment of self-direction leads to assessment of adjustment.

Although these differences may appear minor or useless in interpreting Abdellah's theory, they could have an impact on the nurse's approach to patient care. Ask yourself if the following statements are correct:

> In the circular model the nurse *continually* seeks to identify a nursing problem in which she can assist a patient in meeting an unmet need.

> In the nondirectional model the nurse knows she must deal with a patient's need from a *framework* of the patient's ability to self-direct and adjust to a solution.

> In the linear model the nurse knows that unmet needs *lead* her to question the patient's ability to self-direct and adjust to a given situation.

All of the above statements are correct. Circular models reflect a continuous process, nondirectional models give a general framework in which to see the world with no sense of direction, and linear models provide a direction and lead the thinking process (see Chapter 2). You need to recognize that all the models speak to the same concepts—nursing problems, needs, and so on. It is the interplay or relationship between these concepts that differ.

Like Henderson, Abdellah does identify specific nursing problems that closely relate to the previous theories discussed in this chapter. These were developed in 1953 in order to develop a typology/classification system for nursing problems. The basic criteria for their development recognized that the major physical needs and emotional problems were similar among patients, and rehabilitative measures offered by nursing stemmed from similar nursing problems.

The following represent Abdellah's list of twenty-one nursing problems by categories. The major concepts are italicized.

Basic Problems:
1. To maintain good *hygiene* and physical *comfort.*
2. To promote optimal *activity,* exercise, rest, and sleep.
3. To promote *safety* through the prevention of accident, injury, or other trauma, and through the prevention of the spread of infection.
4. To maintain good *body mechanics* and prevent and correct deformities.

Sustenal and Care:
5. To facilitate the maintenance of a supply of *oxygen* to all body cells.
6. To facilitate the maintenance of *nutrition* to all body cells.
7. To facilitate the maintenance of *elimination.*
8. To facilitate the maintenance of *fluid* and electrolyte balance.
9. To recognize the *physiological response* of the body to disease conditions—pathological, physiological, and compensatory.
10. To facilitate the maintenance of *regulatory mechanisms* and functions.
11. To facilitate the maintenace of *sensory function.*

Remedial-Psychological:
12. To identify and accept positive and negative expressions, *feelings,* and reactions.
13. To identify and accept the interrelatedness of *emotions* and organic illness.
14. To facilitate the maintenance of effective verbal and nonverbal *communication.*
15. To promote the development of productive *interpersonal relationships.*

16. To facilitate progress toward achievement of personal *spiritual goals.*
17. To create and/or maintain a *therapeutic environment.*
18. To facilitate *awareness of self* as an individual with varying physical, emotional, and developmental needs.

Restorative Care:

19. To accept the *optimum* possible *goals* in light of limitations, physical and emotional.
20. To use *community resources* as an aid in resolving problems arising from illness.
21. To understand the role of *social problems* as influencing factors in the cause of illness.

The nursing problems described in Abdellah and Levine's *Better Patient Care Through Nursing Research* are related to a condition and/or situation in which the nurse can be of assistance. They are broken down into four categories: basic health problems common to all patients, sustenal care needs which relate to physiological body processes, remedial care needs generally related to emotional and interpersonal problems, and restorative care needs involving individual and community problems.

The *basic health* problems are intrinsic to the major functions as identified at that time, at least by the nurses caring for the hospitalized patient. They constitute the care of an acute-care patient, such as a postoperative patient, who requires assistance with hygiene, needs rest and sleep, must be protected against injury and infection, and needs to be assisted to move in and out of bed. Abdellah, like Henderson, focuses on what is basic or unique to nursing in caring for patients. Admittedly, these basic health problems are needs of the well and ill whether they are in a hospital, in a clinic, or at home. Yet for the most part individuals who are not acutely or chronically ill can care for their own basic needs without assistance.

The *sustenal care* needs encompass the physiological needs. As recognized by Maslow, they are largely pathophysiological in nature and are relatively overt, dealing with observations of the patient's color, skin, and elimination patterns. There is a strong relationship between the recognition of the sustenal problems and the nurse's monitoring of the basic health problems. For example, a patient who is having difficulty maintaining adequate nutrition (6) would need careful attention to hygiene and comfort to prevent bed sores and physical discomfort.

The *remedial care* needs involve problems that are basically covert and require indirect methods for assessment, such as reflecting, listening, and questioning. These largely relate to Maslow's belonging and love needs and Henderson's needs relating to worship, communication, and work. Again, the health status of a patient in relation to his basic and sustenal problems strongly influences remedial or psychological needs. Negative feelings do evolve from a lack of physical comfort or inability to get oxygen.

The last grouping of nursing problems, the *restorative* problems, relate to the impact that the community, its resources, and its problems have on an individual. This emphasizes the rehabilitative aspect of nursing problems, such as dealing with a patient who has limited physical or emotional ability and requires community resources to achieve the highest level of health. Abdellah brings in the public health emphasis on social problems as they relate to illness. This differs from the approaches of Henderson and of the non-nursing theorists Murray and Maslow.

This classification system has a hierarchical order like Henderson's and Maslow's. It is consistent with the need theories that we have discussed thus far in that the physiological needs are primary, the emotional needs generally follow, and sociological needs, if mentioned, are last. This system compartmentalizes individuals, yet it attempts to show relationships between one category and another by emphasizing that an individual can have multiple problems or unmet needs at the same time in several categories.

Application to Nursing Process

The use of the nursing process in relation to the Abdellah categories is reviewed in Table 5-8. Examples reflect a multitude of possible patient situations and only speak to one or two problems in each category. Using this approach requires that the nurse be able to classify all assessment data into Abdellah's categories.

Evaluation

The major concept is *nursing problems,* which is defined as a condition in which the nurse can assist individuals or groups. The characteristics/criteria for classifying problems are enumerated, with twenty-one separate problems under four categories. Thus, there is confusion and lack of clarity as to what constitutes a problem or condition; however, Abdellah does attempt, as Murray does, to delineate specific criteria on which to focus. The criteria within the basic,

Table 5-8

Incorporation of Abdellah's Problems
and the Nursing Process

Categories of Problems	Assessment Data	Nursing Diagnosis	Plan	Implementation	Evaluation
Basic problems	Note ability to care for own personal hygiene; review sleep and rest patterns.	Inability to bathe self and rest adequately.	Identify measures necessary to maintain good hygiene and get rest; prevent skin breakdown.	Bathe patient. Create an environment conducive to rest.	Monitor skin condition and amount of rest patient is getting.
Sustenal care need	Review eating and elimination habits.	Poor nutrition.	Facilitate adequate nutrition.	Teach patient about the need for an adequate diet.	Reassess patient's intake of food and bowel habits.
Remedial	Observe ability to adapt to the hospital environment.	Difficulty relating to other patients in the room.	Facilitate communication between patients in a non-threatening way.	Discuss patient's feelings about the other patients in the room.	Reassess patient's adjustment to the other patients.
Restorative	Assess knowledge of resources available to assist patient prior to discharge.	Lack of information about community resources.	Communicate needed information.	Teach and inform patient about the agencies available to assist him.	Identify whether the patient understands what is available.

sustenal, and restorative care problems are best understood through inference (see Chapter 2). The behavioral or psychological areas of remedial care are more abstract and harder to understand. The following is useful in understanding the differences in the categories and problems in terms of their being empirical or abstract (see pp. 23). The major theme in the listing is utilized to demonstrate the point. This is the author's interpretation and not Abdellah's.

Empirical	Inferential	Abstract
	Hygiene state	Comfort
	Activity	Physiological response
	Safety	Feelings
	Body mechanics	Emotions
Rate of breathing	Oxygen level	Communication
(oxygen intake)	Nutrition	Interpersonal
	Fluid	Spiritual
	Elimination	Environment
	Regulatory mechanisms	Self-awareness
	Sensory functions	Optimum goals
	Specific resources	Social problems
	(such as money)	

The empirical concepts are identified in an attempt to show that a problem related to oxygen can be deduced by focusing on the rate of breathing, and a specific community resource can be extracted from social problems. In reality there are no *genuine* empirical concepts, but the nurse tends to break those that are abstract down to inferential or empirical concepts so that they can be useful. For example, the abstract concept of *interpersonal* may mean to one nurse that the patient has problems relating to others or accepting his need to have relationships. Another nurse may interpret *interpersonal* to mean what the first nurse understood, in addition to the idea of respecting the individual's (patient's in relation to others) need for a sense of worth and dignity. The interpretation could go on and on. For the most part, the concepts within this theory are relatively abstract and inferential, and each nurse in practice tends to develop her own interpretations of specific meanings. From a general interpretation, these concepts appear to be logical and to relate well to nursing, at least as it was practiced during the 1950s and early 1960s. In addition, the problems that relate to human needs are conceptual, in agreement with previous writers such as Maslow and Henderson.

Abdellah presents no model of her own. Some theorists, such as

King and Roy, do, as you will see later. Thus, in developing models, one must interpret Abdellah's meaning of the concepts and their relationship. Propositions that could be developed and tested for validity are only extracted and interpreted from Abdellah's writing; they are not her own. Although, as you will see, there is a lack of clarity of the concepts in all nursing theories, this theory does facilitate nursing by describing and explaining the patient situation. Its power to predict is questionable unless one were dealing with a very specific problem, such as, for example, a lack of fluid, and one administered liquids and saw dehydration disappear. Given most of the inferential and abstract concepts identified, little or no real prediction is possible using this theory except in the physiological area, which really belongs to the sciences of physiology and medicine.

IDA JEAN ORLANDO: DESCRIPTION OF THE THEORY

Orlando's theory, which evolved at about the same time as Abdellah's, also focuses on differentiating medicine from nursing. She states that nursing offers whatever help patients may require for their needs to be met. *Need* is defined as a requirement of the patient. In her book, *The Dynamic Nurse-Patient Relationship,* she adds that needs are to be met "for his physical and mental comfort to be assured as far as possible while he is undergoing some form of medical treatment or supervision" (p. 5). She identifies, as do Abdellah and Henderson, that it is when patients cannot deal with what they need or when they cannot carry out the prescribed treatment alone that nursing, which is situationally defined, assists the patient. When the patient has a need supplied and the immediate distress is relieved or diminished, a sense of adequacy or well-being can result.

The major concepts in Orlando's definition of nursing are *immediate need, physical and mental comfort, distress, adequacy,* and *well-being.* These concepts are not clearly defined and are fairly abstract. One can assume that Orlando was aware of Murray's, Maslow's, and Henderson's writings and built on their ideas. As you will understand later, Orlando's basic contribution focuses on how nurses process information rather than on specific needs or on the content of nursing. Orlando does not define the concepts, but they can be interpreted within the framework of general usage. The common language meaning, although useful, is not fully adequate to specifically guide nursing practice. Definitions used by professionals should be specific and have clarity within the discipline.

Orlando does not adequately relate to the four basic concepts in nursing (health, nursing, human, and environment). *Humans* have the characteristics of having needs and dealing with comfort/discomfort in stressful situations. Apparently, *health* is a state of comfort—feelings of adequacy and well-being. The *environment* is viewed as affecting human beings in terms of their immediate needs. *Nursing* is more fully explained in terms of the nursing process rather than in terms of the individual needs approach taken by Henderson and Abdellah.

The nursing process is viewed as the interaction between the *behavior* of the patient, the *reaction* of the nurse, and the nursing *actions* designed to meet the patient's immediate need.

Models and Application to the Nursing Process

Orlando does not specifically model her theory, but she offers some propositions/assumptions that could influence the development of a model. It may be useful to identify some assumptions that may be inherent in her theory, and then within the context of the identified concepts develop possible models for clarity. The linear and directional approach to theory development would be used (see Chapter 3), which supports movement back and forth within the nursing process—assessment, diagnosis, plan, reassessment, rediagnosis, replan, and implementation, with many other possible combinations.

Some propositions inherent in Orlando's theory are discussed in her book. Those related to behavior are as follows:

Observations that are shared and explored with a patient are immediately useful in meeting the individual's needs if they exist at that time.

Observations of the nurse are indirect or direct. *Indirect knowledge* is any information that is derived from a source other than the patient, such as data obtained from the family or from nursing service personnel. *Direct knowledge* is any perception, thought, or feeling the nurse has from her experiences in observing the patient behavior.

The behavior of the patient may be perceived from nonverbal motor expression, such as eating, and physiological manifestations, such as respiration and verbal behavior.

Those related to nurses' *reactions* are as follows:

Nurses' reactions are based on the perception of the behavior of the patient, the thoughts that evolve from that perception, and the feelings experienced by the nurse to those perceptions and thoughts.

Unless the nurse's reaction to the patient is validated it should not be assumed to be correct.

The following relates to the nurse's *activity*: nursing actions are either *deliberative,* in which they meet the immediate need of the patient, or *automatic,* in which they are not intended to meet the patient's immediate need, such as those actions ordered by the physician.

The model shown in Figure 5-8 attempts to incorporate the major concepts in the definition which Orlando's view of the nursing process developed from the above propositions in relation to a deliberative action rather than an automatic action. It is compared to the nursing process on the right.

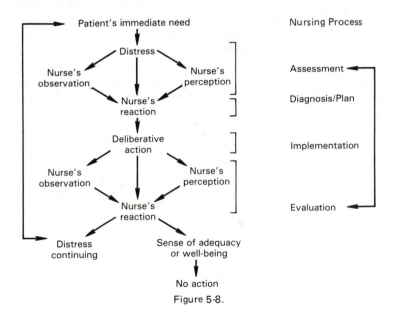

Figure 5-8.

From the model, which is basically linear, the following statement, which integrates Orlando's concepts and propositions, seems valid:

The patient's immediate need arises from a state of distress, causing the nurse to react to her observations and perceptions. This leads to a deliberative action on the part of the nurse (in terms of the patient's identified need). Such an action again causes the nurse to observe and react in order to determine whether a sense of adequacy and well-being has been achieved. The process continues until the immediate distress is gone.

In their book *Concept Formalization in Nursing Process and Product* (p. 59), the Nursing Development Conference Group offers another model, shown in Figure 5-9. Again, because the theorist did not offer a model, numerous interpretations are expected.

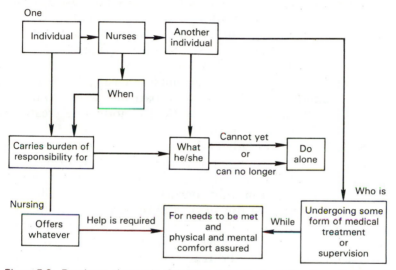

Figure 5-9. Dominant themes in Orlando's concept of nursing; formalization of nurse as responsible agent in relation to patient agency theme. From Nursing Development Conference Group, *Concept Formalization in Nursing, Process and Product,* p. 59. Little Brown & Co., 1973.

The model shown in Figure 5-9 is both similar to and different from the previous one in many ways. The nurse is central to both models, as is the emphasis on or identification of needs to be met in order to achieve a state of comfort/well-being. The latter model focuses much more on the individual and what he can, or can no longer, do alone. It also relates to the time at which the action is taken rather than directly identifying the immediate nature of the need. While the first model reflects the deliberative action and the nurse's reactions, observations, and perceptions, the latter model deals with the automatic activities involved in identifying the needs to be met in relation to the medical treatment. Each interpretation would produce similarities and differences in the nurse's approach to the patient's needs. In the initial model, the nurse would be fully aware that her reactions are due to her observations and perceptions concerning the patient's needs, which could strongly influence her actions; this would not be a significant factor in the second model. For example, a nurse caring for a patient who had had a myocardial infarction would need to understand that her observations and perceptions might be influenced by her own personal experiences. Orlando emphasizes that such observations must be validated with the patient before an action takes place, which makes sense based on this model. In the model shown in Figure 5-9, the nurse would focus on the individual and on her responsibility as related to what the patient cannot yet do alone or can no longer do alone. Admittedly, if a patient needed fluids or oxygen, both models would no doubt lead to the administration of fluid and oxygen in some form. In other situations, however, such as the case of a patient experiencing discomfort, different actions might evolve. The nurse focusing on what the patient can or cannot do might assess the patient's ability to deal with the discomfort. Regardless of the particular model one creates from Orlando's theory, an action is warranted based on needs.

Table 5-9 integrates Orlando's version of the nursing process in a situation that she developed for discussion. Since the situation lacks details, especially about what happened after the second nurse entered the scene, one can only speculate about the possibilities, as was done in the Table. In the automatic response of the first nurse, there was no real analysis of observations and perceptions—neither hers nor the patient's. She viewed the activity as merely following the physician's orders. She did react, but probably with no real objective conscious effort. The second nurse, acting in a more deliberative manner, was apparently aware of the first nurse's reaction and focused on the patient's perception of the situation in order to develop her own set of observations and perceptions to direct her actions. Orlando is quick to remind the nurse that unless we deal with "ineffective" behavior, we cannot assist the patient.

Evaluation

The major focus of Orlando's theory is on the nurse's reaction to the patient's behavior in terms of his immediate need. *Perception* thus becomes a key concept, but it is not well developed. The goal of achieving comfort, adequacy, and well-being is interesting, but ways in which to measure such concepts are not defined. One is left with very little understanding of individuals and of the characteristics they

Table 5-9

Incorporation of Orlando's Model*
with the Nursing Process, Based
on a Situation Presented by Orlando

Situation: A Patient Refuses a Pill: As the nurse was about to hand a patient a dicumarol tablet, she said, "I have a pill for you." The patient said, "Let's see it." The nurse placed the pill within the patient's view. "You're crazy; I'm not going to take that." The nurse flushed and left the room. Another nurse asked the patient, "Can you tell me why you won't take your pill?" "Because I took one just a minute ago." "Who gave it to you?" "Myself—I brought my own dicumarol with me. It was time to take it and I did." (Orlando, I.J. *The Dynamic Nurse-Patient Relationship: Function, Process and Principles.*)

Immediate Need	Assessment		Diagnosis	Plan	Implementation	Evaluation
	Nurse observation	*Nurse perception*				
Administration of medication (automatic activity)—first nurse	Need for medication; Refusal to take medication	Uncooperative; hostile patient reaction	Refusal to take medication	Ask someone else to give the medication	Refuse to administer the medication	Medication not given by herself —unsuccessful
Reduction of confusion about taking medication (deliberative action)—second nurse	Patient has reasons for refusal	Patient is cooperative since she knows she only needs one dose of this medication	Patient is unaware of nurse's role in giving medication and insecure about whether nurse will give medicine	Explain to the patient the value of having the nurse administer the medication to her	Offer medication on schedule	See whether the patient accepts medication from nurse

*Situation is taken from Orlando. The use of the nursing process is original.

manifest. *Health* as a concept apparently relates to *well-being*. *Environment* receives little or no attention except possibly through indirect knowledge. Because Orlando did not develop a model, and because the concepts are not only abstract but also not defined, the content of the theory is weak. Thus the theory at best describes a nursing situation in which the nurse must process information. There is little explanation or predictive power to the theory. Again its major strength is that it provides the nurse with a framework with which to view patients from a nursing perspective rather than from a medical-disease orientation.

ERNESTINE WIEDENBACH:
DESCRIPTION OF THE THEORY

In *Clinical Nursing: A Helping Art,* Wiedenbach describes nursing as a practice in relation to *individuals* who have a *need of help* influenced by a behavioral *stimulus* based on a *philosophy* and oriented toward a specific *purpose* (p. 11). Wiedenbach does not list a set of needs, but she defines *need* as anything the individual requires to maintain and sustain himself comfortably or capably in a situation. *Help* is defined as an action or measure enabling the individual to overcome whatever interferes with his ability to function. Wiedenbach states that when the need for help is met, the individual has potential for restoring or extending his ability to cope with the demands of any situation. Thus the specific purpose of nursing becomes that of assisting patients to *cope.* Coping is viewed as an intrinsic quality that continuously develops throughout life.

Humans are described as functional beings who grow and develop, communicate, and have physical structures, physiological systems, and nervous systems with which they think, interpret, recall, and experience life. If any of these characteristics is impaired or blocked from usage by a stimulus, the individual will have difficulty coping and distress will occur.

Wiedenbach states that the nurse's thoughts and feelings are the most significant portion of the nurse's practice, because they determine the effect of her overt acts on the patient. Nursing blends thoughts, feelings, and overt actions in practice. The similarities between Orlando and Wiedenbach should be fairly evident at this point. The focus on needs, distress, and the nurse's reaction to the patient's behavior are similar. Basic to the theory is the recognition that clinical nursing is composed of four interacting components: philosophy, purpose, practice, and art. These components influence the nurse's ability and responsibility to conserve life and promote health.

Table 5-10 identifies the interlocking components and explains their meanings and the assumptions developed by Wiedenbach. Most of the assumptions explain *human beings* and the practice of *nursing*. The *environment* is identified as that which affects the individual's ability to respond to obstacles. *Health* as a concept is not really identified unless one interprets the individual's lack of the need for help as a state of health. *Nursing* is central to the theory, as it is in Orlando's, and the meeting of needs gives the nurse direction.

Table 5-10

Integrating actions	Wiedenbach's Major Concepts	Nursing Process

	Nurse's
	    philosophy
	    sensation
	    perception
	    validation of assumptions
	        with patient
	Individual's characteristics
	    self-help
	    identification of needs
		Assessment by both nurse
		    and patient

	Assumptions—need for help	Nursing diagnosis
	Planning and designing care with patient	Planning

Goal-directed
and deliberative
insight decision making
	Ministrative by providing
	    help
	Coordination of service
	    with other members
	    of the health team
		Implementation

	Validation that help resulted
	    in patient's ability to
	    function
		Evaluation

Models

Wiedenbach speaks of seven levels of awareness within a reality situation. The realities of the situation identify the nurse as the agent, the patient as the recipient of care, the goal, the measure to attain the goal, and the general framework or environment involved.

Nursing is practiced. The *realities* could be modeled as shown, in support of the statement that the nurse works with the patient to achieve a goal through the use of her knowledge and resources within the context of the environment.

Agent	Recipient	To achieve a goal	Means or process
Nurse	Patient	Nursing action	Application of knowledge and resources

The levels of awareness range from those that are intuitive (based on a sensation, a perception, or an assumption) to those that are voluntary and cognitive (like realization through validation, insight through new information, design, or planning, and responsible decision making). If we place the levels on a continuum, with the most professional approach on the right, it looks like this:

Levels of Awareness

Least Cognitive and Reactive; More Natural						*Most Deliberative and Professional*
Sensa-tion	*Percep-tion*	*Assump-tion*	*Vali-dates*	*Increased*	*Planning*	*Decision Making*
based on percep-tion	related to an inter-preta-tion of a sen-sory impres-sion	more im-pulsive action	assump-tion in reality (realiza-tion)	insight through informa-tion	and de-signing with pa-tient	thought and re-spon-sible action

A nurse uses all these approaches depending on the situation in which she finds herself and the patient. For example, if a patient needs help reaching a glass of water, the nurse would probably react in terms of her perception of the situation and assume the patient wants a drink. On the other hand, if a patient refuses to take an important medication, increased insight, information, and planning would be essential. In a sense, the least cognitive behaviors are those that we all use—habits. We think about them very little, and they are usually functional for us. On the other hand, when we are involved in making an important decision, such as deciding which job to take, we use a more deliberative approach in planning and carrying out a course of action.

Placing the concepts identified within the seven levels of awareness within the realities previously modeled and the interlocking components, we could visualize the unified model (Fig. 5-10) representing these major themes.

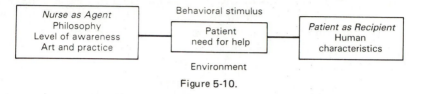

Figure 5-10.

The following assumptions support Wiedenbach's theory and reflect the developed model: The nurse as agent and the patient as recipient of care are focusing on the patient's need for help influenced by the behavioral stimulus and the environment. The nurse is affected by her philosophy, level of awareness, and approach to the art and practice of nursing. The patient has human characteristics which affect his need for help.

Within Wiedenbach's 1969 revised theory (the original writing was in 1964) is an emphasis on a *prescription* that directs the activity. This prescription involves voluntary cognitive action on the part of the nurse and patient in an agreed-upon action, either a nurse-directed activity or a patient-directed activity. This is supported within the model presented, because the need for help is placed central to both the nurse and patient. Nurse theorists are increasingly taking the position that patients need to participate in the process of making decisions about their care and to meet their own needs if possible.

Application to Nursing Process

The use of Wiedenbach's theory provides the nurse with a systematic way of thinking, or, better still, a nursing frame of reference for practice. Thus, it is somewhat difficult to compare her model to the nursing process. In so doing, one loses some of her intent and may easily misinterpret her nursing approach. Since the nursing process is utilized to such a large extent, however, some relationship is helpful. Review the relationship shown in Table 5-10, realizing that the concepts in the nursing process do not exactly fit Wiedenbach's, and that the most deliberative and professional approach is used (versus the reactive or sensory approach).

Some of Wiedenbach's major emphases—the integration of actions and the recognition of what is involved in the assessment data—give clarity to the nursing process. Included in the gathering of information or assessment data are the nurse's philosophy of human beings and her perceptions of the situation as related to the behavior/characteristics of the individual in relation to the need for help. The integrating actions should not be isolated in any one step of the nursing process but should be included in each and every step. The entire nurse-patient interaction is to be goal directed and deliberative, as influenced by the nurse's insight into the situation in which the nurse and the patient finds themselves. Decision making is a constant phenomenon influencing each step of the process.

With the focus on the nurse and the decision-making process, review the following patient situation.

SITUATION

Miss Hernandez, age 18, and her family have just entered the prenatal clinic. She is three months pregnant and has come for her initial checkup with Miss Bauer, a nurse midwife. Miss Hernandez is not sure if she intends to keep the child. Her physical condition appears excellent, and her parents are supportive of her needs. The stimulus for her care is her decision that she is probably pregnant.

Miss Bauer has worked with unwed mothers and believes that if possible they should have and keep their children. In assessing Miss Hernandez, she discusses her feelings about pregnancy and about the child. During the assessment Miss Hernandez expresses her need for help in deciding what she will do. She is aware that if she is to have an abortion, she must have it done soon. Miss Bauer does a complete physical assessment and finds Miss Hernandez in an excellent state of health. Her greatest need seems to be for information so that she can understand the implications of the decisions she will make.

At this point, the nursing process would be utilized as follows:

Assessment. The nurse's philosophy and her perception of the situation will have a strong impact on the individual's decision unless she makes a *deliberate* and conscious effort to neutralize her beliefs. The nurse understands that human beings basically have a reverence for life but that Miss Hernandez as an individual has a right to make her own decision.

Diagnosis. Information about her initial physical examination; need for help in the form of information and the expression of feelings; normal prenatal course.

Plan. Design an approach to provide information in an objective manner. Coordinate any assistance she may need from other health care professionals.

Implementation. Refer to counselor and/or parenting classes after providing information about pregnancy.

Information Evaluation. Validate the information and/or referral; assist Miss Hernandez in making a decision.

From this limited presentation it is evident that Wiedenbach gives nursing a way of incorporating beliefs with deliberative action that is taken on a conscious level. Admittedly, a great deal more could have been identified, especially in the assessment phase. For example, all of the data gathered from a physical examination, from the interaction with her parents, and from the statements made by Miss Hernandez would be included. Wiedenbach's theory and its use here could make a major difference in the outcome of nursing care. Simply approaching Miss Hernandez through the use of the nursing process and focusing on her physical needs might create different outcomes.

Evaluation

Wiedenbach's concepts in relation to human beings, environment, and health are not developed. Her focus on nursing as a process in relation to the need for help does have some clarity, because she explains in detail the method nurses should use in making decisions. The assumptions about human nature are basically philosophical and are generally accepted as truths without research data to validate them. For example, the assumption that an individual's behavior is the best he can do at a given time is difficult to research, since *best* is hard to define or evaluate. Other assumptions, such as the assumption that practice requires knowledge, judgment, and skill on the part of the nurse, could be researched by measuring the quality of care that would be provided by nurses with different levels of knowledge or education.

There is vagueness within Wiedenbach's theory, which is summarized in Table 5-11, especially in relation to the goal of care. The

Table 5-11

Summary of Wiedenbach's Theory

Interlocking Components	Meaning	Assumptions (Weidenbach's)
Philosophy of nurse	Nurse's belief, code of conduct, personal characteristics, and uniqueness developed from her culture. Basic concepts include reverence for the gift of life; respect for the dignity, worth, autonomy, and individuality of human beings; and the resolution to act dynamically in relation to one's beliefs.	Each human being is endowed with unique potential to develop within himself resources which enable him to maintain and sustain himself. The human being basically strives toward self-direction and relative independence and desires not only to make best use of his capabilities and potentialities but to fulfill his responsibilities. Self-awareness and self-acceptance are essential to the individual's sense of integrity and self-worth. Whatever the individual does represents his best judgment at the moment of his doing it.
Purpose of clinical nursing	To facilitate the individual's efforts to overcome the obstacles that are interfering with the ability to respond capably to demands being made by a condition, environment, situation, and time.	The helping measure is influenced by the following: Nervous system responds to the individual's perceptions of the helping act, the environment, memories, association, anticipation. Individuals are physically, physiologically, and psychologically reacting beings.
Practice	Goal directed, deliberatively carried out, and patient-centered approach in relation to a need for help.	Practice requires knowledge, judgment, and skills on the part of the nurse. The patient's perception of his condition or situation is the result of his background of experience and understanding (his frame of reference).

Consists of four components: identification, ministration, validation, and coordination of resources

Identification includes assessing whether the patient has a need, recognizes it, and has the ability to meet

Ministration involves providing the help.

Validation is evidence that the help resulted in the patient's ability to function.

Coordination is integrating her service with the service of others in the health team through reporting, consulting and conferring.

Art

Application of knowledge and skill to achieve goal directed practice based on a one-to-one relationship with the patient's immediate situation.

The nurse can assess the individuality of the patient in terms of what he is experiencing.

The greater the resources, the greater the potential for giving effective care.

Evidence for validation can be gained from the patient's behavior.

Total medical care is a cooperative venture for the benefit of the patient.

The helping process triggered by a stimulus, which is the patient's behavior.

The helping process contains the feelings and perceptions of the nurse as related to her expectations about the patient's behavior.

Nursing actions are *natural* when guided by the nurse's immediate perception of the patient's behavior. Actions are *reactionary* when the nurse responds spontaneously using the feelings that have been evoked by her perception of the patient's behavior.

Deliberative action is interaction directed toward fulfillment of an explicit purpose; it includes information, analysis, and judgment.

level of need for help is not discussed in any depth, yet it affects the deliberative process of nursing. The concept *nursing* is explained from multiple frameworks—philosophy, levels of awareness, prescriptive process and actions, the realities of the situation—which are not clearly integrated within a single framework for use and would lead the nurse in different directions. Would the nurse be influenced more by her perception, the patient's reality, the environment, or the need for help? This makes the theory less than easy to understand and thus to use. A theory such as this which focuses on process orientation would probably be more effective with one client than would one that focuses on content, such as Henderson's or Abdellah's. The integration of Henderson's and Abdellah's specifically identified needs and Wiedenbach's decision-making process would be more fruitful. At the end of this chapter, this integration will be further discussed.

DOROTHEA E. OREM: DESCRIPTION OF THE THEORY

In her text *Nursing: Concepts of Practice,* Orem describes her theory, the central assumption of which relates to the fact that people who are subject to health-related or health-derived limitations become incapable of providing independently for their own self-care needs (p. 27). The three major concepts of her theory are *self-care, self-care deficits,* and *nursing systems. Self-care* relates to regulating structural integrity, human functioning, and development, and is continuous throughout life. *Self-care deficits* are predictive of a nursing requirement and give a focus to nursing to explain when and why it is necessary. (This is actually the frame of reference for nursing.) *Nursing systems* is the approach to practice by which the nurse acts in relation to the patient's self-care needs and deficits. Orem provides a model (Fig. 5-11) relating these major concepts in her text (p. 24).

Models

The model appears to be both circular and linear. Each concept leads to another. Self-care → therapeutic self-care demand → nursing capabilities → self-care capabilities → self-care. The major focus is linear. The degree of therapeutic self-care demand as related to the self-care capabilities may provide for a deficit relationship in which nursing capabilities become necessary.

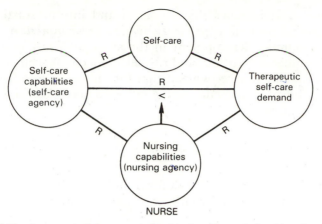

Figure 5-11. A conceptual framework for nursing (R = relationship; < = deficit relationship, current or projected). From Dorothy E. Orem, *Nursing: Concepts of Practice.* 2nd Edition, 1980, McGraw Hill, New York, p. 24.

Another way of developing this model which would reflect the same relationship between the concepts is shown in Figure 5-12.

Within a given situation, individuals have self-care needs and demands; their capability of meeting these needs influences whether nursing is needed or not. If the demand or need is greater than the individual's ability to meet it, a deficit situation requiring nursing results. If the individual is capable of meeting his own needs, no nursing action is necessary, and the individual is responsible for himself.

In relation to the four major concepts, Orem's major contribution relates to understanding *nursing* and *individuals* (humans) in relation to their self-care needs. As was the case with Wiedenbach's theory, the role of the nurse is primary within this theory; as in Henderson's and Abdellah's theories, the identification of specific needs is offered. Thus, it will become increasingly evident that Orem followed the approach offered by the previously presented need theorists.

The concept of *health* strongly relates to self-care and sustaining life processes, maintaining integrating functioning, preventing and regulating disease and disability, and promoting normal growth and

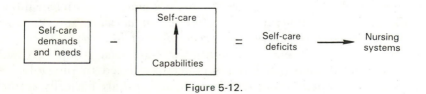

Figure 5-12.

development. It includes psychological and interpersonal social aspects of living as well as physical health. *Environment* is viewed as facilitating human development in the areas of forming or changing attitudes, values, creativity, and the self-concept as well as the physical development. It is recognized that the environment affects the individual's ability to provide for his self-care needs, as is most evident in the hospital.

Application to Nursing Process

The following major assumptions/propositions must be accepted in order to utilize Orem's theory for practice:

Self-care activities and needs represent the major focus of the practice of nursing.

The individual's ability to meet self-care needs is influenced by developmental level, life experiences, cultural orientation, health, and available resources.

Orem identifies multiple propositions that give greater clarity to the major propositions for practice. These propositions are offered with models and some implications for practice. Again, theory is the knowledge we need in order to process information about patients. In this case the models are developed from the propositions offered (Table 5-12), even though one usually develops models before propositions in reviewing and developing theories (see Chapter 2).

These models, as developed, provide a way of looking at any situation in which a nurse interacts with a patient. As a matter of fact, all these models, in addition to many other propositions and models Orem developed that are not stated here, must all be used at the same time; this gives a comprehensive view of nursing practice.

As noted in the third proposition, *self-care requisites* (previously called *requirements* by Orem), which could also be called *self-care needs,* are: *universal, developmental,* and *health deviation.* The universal self-care requisites are very similar to Murray's and Henderson's approaches to basic physiological needs. Universal requisites common to all human beings are the maintenance of sufficient intake of *air, water,* and *food*; adequate *elimination, activity,* and *rest*; *solitude* and social *interaction*; the *prevention* of *hazard*; and the promotion of *normal* human *functioning* within *social* groups. As with the other need theorists, Orem's concepts related to physiological needs like air, water, food, elimination, and rest are basically empirical concepts which are easily identified and researched. The latter three requisites are more abstract and can be understood mostly by inference. Orem provides some criteria in relation to these requisites. For example, the criteria for solitude and social interaction relate to maintaining quality and balance of personal autonomy and enduring social relations, fostering bonds of love and affection, and offering social warmth. Orem explains that her concept of *normal* relates to developing and maintaining a realistic self-concept, fostering human development, promoting integrity of one's structure and functioning, and attending to deviations.

Development requisites are related both to promoting human progress toward a higher level of organization and to preventing conditions that would hinder effective human development. These requisites interrelate with the development of the universal self-care requisite. For example, during the infancy stage a caretaker must provide for the need for safety and love. If these needs are not adequately met, the child will fail to develop. Problems related to social adaptation, educational deprivation, and loss of friends all relate to the universal requisite of social interaction and to the development stage of the individual.

Health deviation requisites stem from the individual's illness, defects, or disabilities, which are identified during the individual's involvement with medical treatment. Normal functioning is not present and the individual seeks medical assistance, usually for a pathological condition. These requisites often involve changes in self-concept, comfort, and life-style. Again these requisites strongly relate to those that are universal and developmental.

Orem identifies two *technologies* which reflect components or approaches to the nursing process—interpersonal and regulatory processes. *Interpersonal technologies* involve communication, interperson and intragroup relations, maintaining therapeutic relationships, and assisting individuals to adapt by meeting their needs. *Regulatory technologies* include maintaining and promoting life processes, regulating psychophysiological functioning, promoting growth and development, and regulating movement and position in space. Thus, these technologies deal with the nursing process from interpersonal as well as from regulation perspectives. The terminology presented by Orem differs somewhat, but the decision-making process is similar. The emphasis here is on self-care needs/requisites and on the nurse as an individual in relation to the interpersonal process. This approach is not unlike Wiedenbach's.

Within the context of the nursing process, Orem provides a conceptual way of understanding a nursing system reflective of an ap-

Table 5-12

Orem's Propositions	Possible Models	Some Implications for Practice
1. Self-care and care of dependents rest on the cultural attainments of cultural attainments of social groups and on the educability of their individual members.	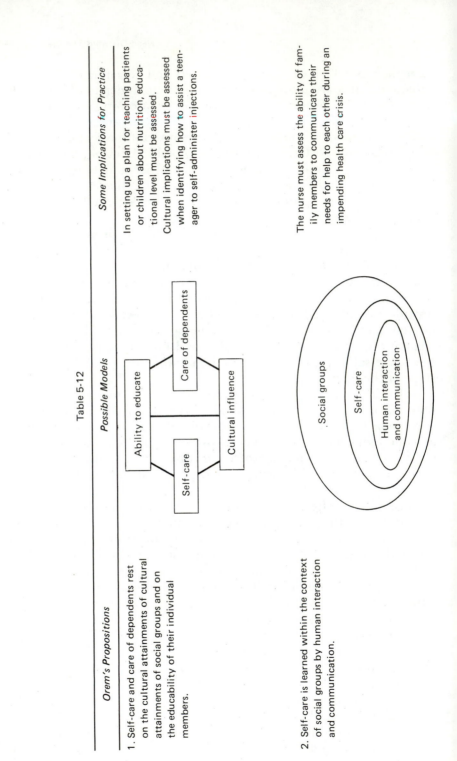	In setting up a plan for teaching patients or children about nutrition, educational level must be assessed. Cultural implications must be assessed when identifying how to assist a teenager to self-administer injections.
2. Self-care is learned within the context of social groups by human interaction and communication.		The nurse must assess the ability of family members to communicate their needs for help to each other during an impending health care crisis.

3. Some requisites (requirements) for self-care are common to all human beings; others are specific to the developmental and health states of individuals.

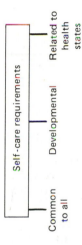

Self-care requirements

Common to all   Developmental   Related to health states

In assessing an individual who is thirsty, the nurse realizes that everyone needs fluids, that children may ask for water as a way of gaining attention, and that postsurgical patients must be observed for dehydration.

4. Nurses and patients act together to allocate the roles of each in the production of patients' self-caring and in the regulation of patients' self-care capabilities.

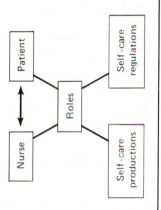

Nurse ⟷ Patient

Roles

Self-care productions   Self-care regulations

In caring for a bedridden patient, the nurse and patient plan together who will perform and meet care needs.

Table 5-13

Orem's Basic Nursing System

Nurse Action	Some Characteristic of Patient	Patient Action
Nurse action ⟶ intense	Patient unable to meet own self-care needs. —state of coma —inability to make decisions *Wholly compensatory system*	Patient action limited
Nurse action ⟶ shared	Patient has limited ability to meet self-care ⟵ needs. —limited knowledge —limited ability to ambulate and to perform manipulative skills *Partly compensatory system*	Patient action shared
Nurse action ⟶ supported	Patient can accomplish self-care. ⟵ —has learned new self-care activities —needs limited help in decision making *Supportive-educative system*	Patient action intensive

Used with permission from Dorothy E. Orem, *Nursing: Concepts of Practice* (New York: McGraw-Hill Book Company, 1971) p. 78.

proach to patient care and analysis that provides for deliberative action as shown in Table 5-13.

The model shown in Figure 5-13 integrates the kind and degree of patient and nursing actions. When the patient has a very limited ability to meet his own universal needs, the nursing actions reflect a greater degree of regulatory technology. Likewise, when the patient requires education and support and can meet his own self-care needs, the nursing action is limited and probably more interpersonal. In reality, there is always some involvement of both the patient and the nurse in any situation. A comatose patient usually will breathe and monitor his intake of air, and a patient who has learned to give himself injections of insulin will seek counseling from the nurse if problems arise. The ultimate goal of practice is to move the patient from a wholly compensatory state to a supportive state if at all possible. Thus education does not occur only during the supportive state. This

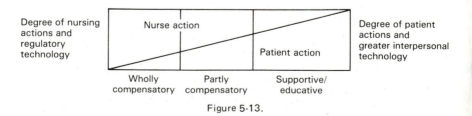

Figure 5-13.

approach should not be viewed simplistically. It reflects merely a tentative analysis of the degree of need for nursing actions.

Application to Nursing Process

Within the context of the model and its terminology, Orem offers a way of calculating the self-care demand. This demand reflects the totality of self-care actions needed to meet the self-care requisites. This can be compared to the nursing process, as shown in Table 5-14.

This approach to the nursing process provides a central focus that is somewhat different from that of the other need theorists. Although the requisites—needs—are the elements of the theory, it is the strong emphasis on self-care that provides a different approach for the nurse. Orlando's approach to the immediate need of the patient with the emphasis on interaction is similar to Orem's, but Orem takes Orlando's idea a major step forward by focusing more on the continuity of care and on the role the nurse plays in providing such care.

Evaluation

The basic concepts of the theory are *self-care* and *nursing systems*. Orem clarifies both these concepts by providing specific criteria on which to focus. *Self-care* is viewed in the context of requisite, universal, developmental, and health deviation, and *nursing systems* from the orientation of the nurse's specific role in supporting the patient's need for self-care. One can assume that her propositions either are viewed as obvious truths or are testable by research. For example, the recognition that individuals need air, water, and food is an obvious, long-validated truth. Propositions that support the position that all patients want to meet their own self-care needs require validation in terms of the particular type of patient, situation, and environment. A resident of a nursing home who has physical and environmental limitations might be less a candidate for self-care than a younger person who is ill at home might be.

The theory is logical and relatively easy to understand. It provides a way of organizing and collecting data and explains the nurse's and the patient's roles in health care. Thus it is a descriptive and explanatory theory, and, with research, could be a predictive theory. It is also congruent with, rather than contradictory to, the other need theories.

Table 5-14

Nursing Process	Focus	Calculation of Self-Care Demand	Some Examples
Assessment	Degree of patient's ability to meet own self-care requisites.	Identify each universal self-care requisite and project potential development and health deviation self-care requisites.	The patient is unable to take fluid postoperatively due to nausea (universal need for fluid due to health deviation requiring surgery).
		Identify internal and external factors that affect the meeting of self-care requisites.	The hospital bed is too high to allow patient to ambulate alone (universal need for activity due to environmental factors).
		Determine ability of patient to meet self-care requisites.	Some patients cannot get out of bed and cannot eliminate without assistance.
Diagnosis	Statement of specific self-care requisites that require nursing actions.	Identify specific self-care demands in relation to patient's ability to meet them.	Inability to meet universal self-care requisites of fluids and mobility; pain and discomfort.
Plan	Development of a therapeutic self-care plan based on a compensatory or educative system.	Design a course of action in relation to the universal self-care demand in relation to the developmental and/or health deviation requisite.	Identify ways in which patient is most comfortable and can reach fluids if desired; support patient when getting out of bed.
		Formulate a total design of self-care action.	
Implementation	Provision of technologies: interpersonal, regulatory, support.	Perform, educate, coordinate, guide, or direct activities to encourage self-care.	Offer fluids; assist patient out of bed.
Evaluation	Review of daily living activities for further deliberative action.	Review with patient and family the prescription for self-care and the progress toward assisting the patient to meet own needs.	Assess patient's ability to hold fluids and get out of bed.

M. LUCILLE KINLEIN:
DESCRIPTION OF THE THEORY

Kinlein's theory, which is described in her book *Independent Nursing Practice and Clients,* is reflective of Orem's theory of self-care. She has modified the concepts within Orem's theory somewhat, but the basic philosophical approach is similar. Inherent within Kinlein's framework is the focus on nursing and how it is different in its knowledge and process from medicine. As Kinlein is an independent nursing practitioner, her writings emerge from the notion that she is accountable to the client and autonomous in the practice of nursing. The following are some of her assumptions (p. 12):

1. The professional nurse cares for the person, not the physician, laboratory staff, and so on. Thus, the individual is the center of the framework. The professional nurse is an extension of the client.
2. The knowledge necessary for the professional nurse relates to meeting individuals' needs rather than making a medical diagnosis or initiating therapy.
3. The greater the medical need, the less need for nursing judgment. Knowing the medical needs does not automatically tell the nurse the nursing needs of the patient.
4. Nursing should be practiced independently and within a framework of nursing theory in order to clarify the role of the professional nurse.
5. Nursing assessment takes time and must be done if professional practice is to occur.

These assumptions highlight Kinlein's emphasis on explaining the practice of professional nursing, as Orem has done, rather than focusing on clarifying the human condition or characteristics, except for the notion of human needs. In separating medicine and nursing, it becomes necessary to clarify the concepts of *health* versus *sickness.* It is possible for the nurse to find the individual "sicker" from a self-care deficit perspective than the physician would from a disease perspective. For example, an individual who is having difficulty with daily personal care following an amputation may be perceived as unhealthy from a nursing point of view. The physician might view the same patient as healthy if the wound has completely healed and the patient is ready for a prosthesis. Nursing's approach to appraising an individual's ability to care for one's own needs is primary to the individual's ability to survive, and is often more difficult to achieve and

more important in relation to a state of health. This is not to minimize the significance of the wound healing; it is only to point out
that stopping where medicine does is not adequate.

Kinlein's approach is to focus on assisting the individual's self-
care practice in regard to one's state of health. Here is the difference
in emphasis between Orem and Kinlein. Kinlein focuses on a state of
health and health goals, while Orem's major emphasis is on needs
that are created as a result of health deviation. In truth, Kinlein's
theory is an extension, not a contradiction, of Orem's theory.

Models

Kinlein models the framework in a somewhat linear way as
shown in Figure 5-14. The following propositions emerge from this
model:

The nurse and the client function together in order to identify
the need for nursing care.

Knowledge and experience are basic to nursing practice.

Nursing care practiced from a framework of self-care assets and
deficits can be more predictable in terms of its outcome.

Client communication and participation focus on self-care assets and deficits.

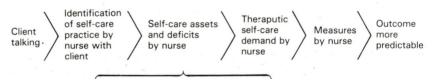

Figure 5-14. Kinlein model. From Kinlein, M. Lucille, *Independent Nursing Practice with
Clients*. p. 24 (used with permission, 1977, Lippincott, Philadelphia, Pa.)

Kinlein identifies this model as her mental construct (*construct*
is the integration of concepts) and views medical care as a part of
nursing care, rather than nursing care as a part of medical care.

The major concepts, similar to those of Orem's theory, are *human self-care needs* and the state of *health*. Health relates to the individual's daily personal care habits. Kinlein asks several questions in
order to find a relationship between self-care and the state of health:

To what extent do pluses and minuses of a person's self-care practices affect the state of health?

If we more clearly understood the self-care practices of human beings, would we be better able to meet self-care needs when there is illness?

These questions are Kinlein's call for further research. A later chapter will discuss the use of research in relation to the various theories proposed.

Applications to Nursing Process

Kinlein's use of the nursing process is similar to Orem's, with the focus on self-care deficits and the role of the nurse. Kinlein stresses that the nurse must refrain from making premature judgments about a client. Thus, the initial contact involves a nurse-client interaction in which the nurse seeks to clarify her understanding of the patient's condition, using her knowledge as a basis for the discussion. Judgments evolve on the part of the nurse when the specific self-care assets and deficits have been identified so that the greater self-care demands can be met through a nursing perception. The nursing process relates in the following way to Kinlein's phases of nursing activities as she identifies them in *Independent Nursing Practice and Clients* (p. 59).

Nursing Process	Kinlein's Phases
Assessment	Greeting the client. Narration by client. Clarification by client.
Diagnosis	Self-care assets and deficits.
Plan	Identification of therapeutic self-care demands.
Implementation	Therapeutic measures.
Evaluation	Identification relating to need for more data. Assessment measures taken in terms of a better health state.

Because Kinlein is an independent nurse practitioner and her focus is on the client, she is continuously thinking about and revising her information with each client contact; the nurse who practices within a hospital might not do this as often. On the other hand, Kinlein's client contacts can extend over a longer period of time and can be based on a greater number of needs, especially informational, emotional, and social needs.

Evaluation

Kinlein's theory provides the professional nurse with a frame of reference (as Kinlein states, a mental construct) with which to practice in relation to a state of health. Thus the concept of *nursing* is well described within her set of assumptions. The model presented defines a clear relationship between the concepts of nurse, client, and self-care. Her questions for research are well developed and, if answered, would provide a stronger theoretical basis for nursing practiced from a need orientation. The theory describes and explains nurse-patient interaction and the focus of practice. The theory relates to the concept of health, but offers little clarity as to its meaning. The environment/society is described by Kinlein basically in terms of the present and potential future status of the health care system. The integration of the four major nursing concepts (human, health, nursing, and environment) is not clear, but we can assume that the basic and only integrating concepts are the client and the nurse.

SUMMARY OF NEED THEORIES

In reviewing each of the need theories from Murray's to Kinlein's, it is evident that there are no basic contradictions; rather, each has a somewhat different frame of reference or way of looking at human needs. The psychological approaches offered by Murray and Maslow enhance the clarity of the nursing theories. Common to all the nursing theories is an attempt to clarify the role and function of professional nursing, especially as differentiated from the practice of medicine. Some nursing theorists, like Henderson, Abdellah, and Orem, offer us the specific needs generally related to the physical, psychological, and social needs of patients. Wiedenbach and Orlando, who do not offer a list of specific needs, apparently accept them as givens needing little explanation.

When the theories are compared, it is evident that some are more closely related than others. Henderson's and Abdellah's themes relate closely to Murray's and Maslow's. Orem's and Kinlein's are closely linked, but Kinlein's is also related to Wiedenbach's in terms of the nursing process. In describing human needs as universal, developmental, and health related, Orem's theory also builds on Henderson's and Murray's. Given certain common assumptions, it may well be that there are more similarities than differences among the theories. One must recognize that the following assumptions may not be as evident in some theories as in others, but none are contradictory within the general framework of need theory.

Assumptions—Nursing Theories and Related Psychological Themes

1. Humans have a set of common needs. The terminology may differ among the theorists, but the meanings are similar, as noted in the following examples:

   Physical needs
   Murray: viscerogenic needs
   Maslow: physiological needs
   Henderson: physical needs, such as breathing and eating
   Abdellah: problems in supplying oxygen, nutrition, etc.
   Orem: universal needs like air, water, food.

   Emotional needs
   Murray: affection between people
   Maslow: belonging and love
   Henderson: communicating emotions and needs
   Abdellah: development of interpersonal relationship
   Orem: solitude and social interaction

   Social needs
   Murray: defense of status; avoiding failure
   Maslow: esteem, desire for reputation
   Henderson: sense of accomplishment
   Abdellah: problems relating to achieving possible goals
   Orem: being normal based on societal standards

According to these theorists, humans can be approached from a common frame of reference—their universal needs. Although Maslow is the only one who clearly identifies a hierarchical order to these needs, it is probable that the other theorists would agree with him. The major differences among these theorists and the way they describe the concept *need* are the details/criteria/characteristics they offer for clarity. Probably Murray attempted to provide the clearest specific descriptions of human needs.

2. Professional nursing's basic responsibility is to meet individuals' needs when they are unable to meet their own, especially during illness.

   All nurse theorists define the nurse's responsibility as helping patients to help themselves if at all possible, with Henderson, Orem, and Kinlein particularly strong on this point. The assessment of the patient includes not only the identification of needs, but also an analysis of whether the patient can provide for his own needs. Teaching the patient or family to care for the identified needs is either stated, as it is in Orem's theory, or implied, as it is in the others.

3. Human needs and the degree to which they are met have an impact on the health status of the individual.

   Generally, the greater the degree to which the nurse must provide for the individual's needs, the lesser the state of health. Health is measured in terms of need satisfaction and degree of nurse participation in care. Healthy individuals can meet their own needs.

4. Need theories basically focus on the ill individual, upon whom the nurse, the family, and the environment have an impact.

   Central to all need theories is the ill individual, whether we call the individual a patient or a client. All theorists focus on the ill individual, except for Kinlein, and she refers to the individual as a client.

5. Utilizing the major concepts offered by the needs themselves will provide a common basis for nursing practice.

   The major concepts are *needs, self-care potential,* and *nursing roles.* The basic model is represented as follows:

$$\frac{\text{Individual's}}{\text{needs}} - \frac{\text{Individual's}}{\text{self-care potential}} = \frac{\text{Nursing role in meeting}}{\text{patient's needs}}$$

The nursing process can effectively be utilized to develop a plan of care from a need framework. The differences between the theorists are relatively minor and would have little real impact on the nurse's implementation of care.

REFERENCES

Abdellah, F.G., I.L. Beland, A. Martin, and R.V. Matheney. *Patient-Centered Approaches to Nursing.* New York: Macmillan, Inc., 1960.

Abdellah, F.G., and E. Levine. *Better Patient Care Through Nursing Research.* New York: Macmillan, Inc., 1968.

Harmer, B., and V. Henderson. *Textbook of Principles and Practice of Nursing,* 5th ed. New York: Macmillan, Inc., 1955.

Henderson, Virginia. *The Nature of Nursing.* New York: Macmillan, Inc., 1966. Idem, *Basic Principles of Nursing Care* (Geneva: International Council of Nurses, 1972).

Kinlein, M.L. *Independent Nursing Practice and Clients.* Philadelphia: J.B. Lippincott Company, 1977.

Maslow, A. *Motivation and Personality.* New York: Harper & Row Publishers, Inc., 1954.

Murray, H. *Explorations in Personality.* New York: Oxford University Press, 1938.

Nursing Development Conference Group. *Concept Formalization in Nursing Process and Product,* 1st ed. Boston: Little, Brown & Company, 1973.

Orem, D.E. *Nursing: Concepts of Practice.* New York: McGraw-Hill Book Company, 1971.

Orlando, I.J. *The Dynamic Nurse-Patient Relationship: Function, Process, and Principles.* New York: G.P. Putnam's Sons, 1961.

Wiedenbach, E. *Clinical Nursing: A Helping Art.* New York: Springer Publishing Company, Inc., 1964.

6

SYSTEMS-ORIENTED THEORIES

INTRODUCTION

The systems-oriented nursing theories emerged during the late six-
ties, about the same time as Robert Chin, Talcott Parsons, and Ludwig von Bertalanffy's writings emerged. Chin wrote about systems
and developmental theory in relation to change. Parsons wrote from
a social-psychological point of view and von Bertalanffy from a biological one. All these writers provide a foundation for a clearer understanding of the systems-oriented nursing theorists. The basic
notion of a systems approach is to view the whole rather than the
parts of a situation: Seeing the parts does not lend itself to understanding the whole. Figure 6-1 provides a frame of reference for this
chapter.

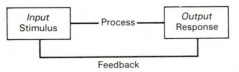

Figure 6-1. Basic systems model.

HISTORICAL DEVELOPMENT

Systems theories were developed after need theories. Within the five-year period between 1967 and 1972 almost all the nursing theorists focused on systems and, as you will note later, built on Chin's, Parsons's, and von Bertalanffy's views of an open system with subsystems that also differ somewhat from each other (Table 6-1).

Table 6-1

Historical Development of Systems Theory

Theory			Major Theme
Health-related theories	Chin	1961	Systems model for practitioners.
	Parsons	1968	General theory of action/personality.
	von Bertalanffy	1968	General systems theory.
	Johnson	1968	A behavioral system with subsystems that can be described and analyzed.
	Rogers	1970	Man is a unified whole within an open system exchanging energy with the environment.
Nursing theories	King	1971	A theory of nursing systems involving perceptions, judgments, actions, reactions, interactions, and transactions leading to goal attainment.
	Neuman	1972	Nursing is a total-person approach in relationship to stress which occurs within and outside the individual.
	Roy	1976	Person is an adaptive system that reacts to stimuli in four modes.

Robert Chin

Chin, who wrote about change, believes that practitioners must have concepts in order to make observations and diagnoses that lead to assumptions about the client-system. His system approach is thought to be universally applicable to human relationships and the physical sciences. Chin visualizes a system by drawing a large circle, as shown in Figure 6-2. Within the circle are elements, variables, and parts with lines which show relationships among them. The lines are viewed as rubber bands or springs that stretch and contract. Outside the circle is the environment.

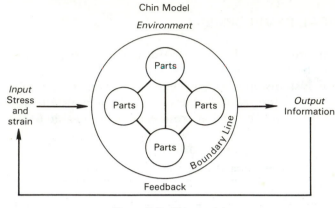

Figure 6-2. Chin model.

The boundary lines assist in separating the inner circle from the environment. Because the parts of the system differ, *stress* and *strain* occur within it as well as outside it. The system is never static nor can it attempt to be; it is constantly changing and attempting to achieve a balanced relationship between the parts, which is called a *steady state.* Since the system is never closed off, inputs and outputs occur around the boundary. A feedback system takes the output/ information about how the parts are doing and turns it into more input. As Chin notes in *The Planning of Change,* organization, interdependency, and integration of the parts are reflective of this system (pp. 297-312).

Talcott Parsons

Parsons, who took some of his ideas from Freud, wrote about a general theory of action, or a theory of personality. *Action* is viewed as a system of organized behavior. A *system* is the structural aspect of the personality of the individual. Every individual is also a unit within a system. There are four primary subsystems within the system: the *personality,* the *behavioral organism,* the *social* and the *cultural* subsystems. The personality is composed of wants, goals, values, and feelings that have been learned through life experiences. The behavior of a living organism is organized, controlled, and based on a cultural, symbolic, coded system. The social subsystem includes all socialization processes, such as one's role, the family, and organizational structures. Each subsystem has an environment, which is an open system; each interchange has output and input with every other. These subsystems articulate with a reference base that is somewhat independent, which reflects a pattern maintenance approach.

This theory assists the individual in developing a meaningful identity system.

Although Parsons's theory is actually reflective of a personality theory, his major concepts provide another base for the understanding of general systems theory. The model shown in Figure 6-3 attempts to explain Parsons's most significant contribution in terms of an open system theory. Since Parsons did not develop a model as such, this symbolic representation is merely interpretive.

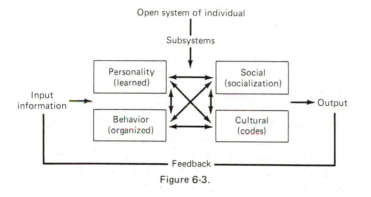

Figure 6-3.

Assumptions that follow the model (Fig. 6-3) and are congruent with Parsons's writing are the following:

1. The individual and his subsystems are within an open system of the environment.
2. An open system is one that has a dynamic, changing interaction with its subsystems. Thus each subsystem interacts with every other, as the lines between them demonstrate.
3. The interaction between each subsystem has input, in the form of information, and output, such as speech, which also could be viewed as information.

Ludwig von Bertalanffy

In his book *General Systems Theory,* von Bertalanffy states that there are general systems laws that apply to different fields of study irrespective of the particular properties of the systems or of the elements involved (p. 37). Thus, he adds to Chin's and Parsons's position concerning a more holistic view of the world. Inclusion of the environment and component common elements provides a generalized frame of reference with which to view the world no matter what the discipline or specific content. It was hoped that general systems theory would integrate the various sciences into a unity of sciences and lead to the integration of scientific education.

Some of the general assumptions developed by von Bertalanffy are as follows:

1. Every living organism is essentially an *open system.*

   An open system involves constant change and interaction with its components, a feedback system, and an open environment. It is the opposite of a static state, or a closed system in which something can be isolated from its environment.

2. An open system tends toward a state of higher organization.

   A feedback mechanism can increase information, and learning can occur. Thus, there is constant forward movement, with increased order and organization.

3. The principle of *equifinality* is reflective of an open system.

   Equifinality means that different conditions can lead to the same final state. Examination of the word leads to the conclusion that different but equal (*equi*) states can lead back to the same final results (*finality*). From a scientific perspective, equifinality allows us to see multiple possibilities rather than just cause and effect, an approach often used by chemists, for example.

4. Organismic processes such as growth are time-independent steady states.

   No equilibrium is achieved here, but a living system with irreversible processes building up and breaking down shows a remarkable ability to be regulated and maintain a steady functioning state.

5. The organization of living organisms or societies has characteristics such as wholeness, growth, differentiation, hierarchical order, dominance, content, and competition.

   Living organisms, according to general systems theory, have common characteristics that facilitate their understanding from a holistic viewpoint. These characteristics can be applied to the total system or subsystems that will be discussed later in reviewing the nursing theories.

6. Within an open system, the organisms can avoid an increase in entropy by maintaining a steady state.

   Entropy occurs when the organization within a system is characterized by a lack of patterning, disorganization, and disorder. As entropy increases, the system breaks down and information is lessened. With increased order and organization of a total system, entropy can be reduced. Entropy implies that matter and energy will become inert and uniform due to disorder and chaos. This very abstract concept is used by nursing theorists and will be discussed again later in this chapter.

Von Bertalanffy clarifies his systems approach by explaining the modern theory of communication. The system is comprised of a receptor which is stimulated, a message, a control apparatus, and an effector which sends a feedback message to the receptor. An adaptation of his model, which is circular, is shown in Figure 6-4.

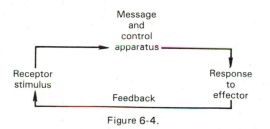

Figure 6-4.

The similarities between the basic systems model presented initially in this chapter and the Chin, Parsons, and von Bertalanffy models should be evident. All utilize stimuli, stress, or information, as input, content, or parts, as subsystems, which are interacting, as process and outputs as responses. Although the concepts within these models are basically abstract, such as stimulus and response, they do have some common characteristics in terms of content and process. The content reflects the idea that within the human environment there are multiple stimuli, such as information being processed, that create a response. This provides a process or a way of thinking about our world that is different from looking at discrete events or things.

In Table 6-2, the basically linear and limited models of the nurse theorists clearly reflect the systems theoretical approach. Each has some form of input, process, and output. The concepts differ in relation to each of these, but the basic idea is the same. Inputs are either stress, perception, matter/energy/information, or stimuli. Processes include some form of integrating human/environment, or subsystems such as adaptive modes, or personal/interpersonal/social systems. Outputs relate with feedback mechanisms to the state of the input concept. Admittedly, differences in abstract concepts do exist between the models, but the thinking process and their relationship to general systems theory is very evident. In utilizing these models

Table 6-2
Basic Components of Systems Models of Nurse Theorists

Theorist	Model (Limited Version)	Conceptual Focus
Johnson	Behavioral system Seven integrated subsystems and balance and dynamic stability Forces and stress → Efficient and effective functioning and adaptation ∨ Ineffective	The goal of nursing is to restore, maintain, or attain behavioral system balance and stability at the highest level.
Rogers	Open system Matter Energy Information → Unitary man and environment as an energy field → Matter Energy Information Change is continuous	Unitary man and the environment are energy fields within an open system which is constantly ex-changing matter, energy, and information. The science of nursing evolves from an open-system framework in order to describe, explain, and predict approaches to nursing care.
King	Perception → Reaction → Interaction → Transaction Goal setting personal interpersonal and social system Feedback	Individuals react and interact with nurses based on their perceptions from a personal, interpersonal, and social system in order to establish a mutual goal.

Neuman

Lines of resistance

Environmental $\longrightarrow$ Energy resources of total $\longrightarrow$ Reconstitution
stress   person

Feedback

Stress within the environment affects the total individual's ability to reconstitute in relation to energy resources and line of resistance.

Roy

Individual

Input stimuli $\longrightarrow$ Adaptive modes $\longrightarrow$ Output
                                              Adaptive or ineffective

Subsystems

Cognitive   Regulative

Feedback

Stimuli affect the individual's adaptive modes which encompass subsystems and the ability to effectively adapt.

for nursing practice, a different frame of reference emerges here than with the need-oriented theories. This approach attempts to use the holistic approach to a greater degree and is a much more all-encompassing way of viewing the interaction between the environment and individuals.

DOROTHY E. JOHNSON: DESCRIPTION OF THE THEORY

Johnson approaches nursing theory from a behavioral systems viewpoint and builds on Chin's theory. She believes that nursing's basic role is to restore, maintain, and obtain a balanced and stable behavioral approach toward social demands, illness, and trauma. She supports the open systems concepts of organization, interdependency, interaction, and integration of parts. The individual's goal is to achieve a behavioral balance and steady state by adjustment and adaptation to certain forces.

The concept of *nursing* is related to supporting a high level of behavior on the part of the individual. The *individual* who has behavioral organization is viewed as the focus of nursing. The *environment* contains forces and stresses that affect behavior, and *health* relates to the ability to maintain an integrated behavioral balance and stability.

Within the behavioral system Johnson makes certain assumptions/propositions that are supportive of the positions of previous writers.

1. The behavioral system is characteristic of the individual's life, with its patterns of purposeful behavior.

    The idea of patterned behavior is significant because it reflects repetitive, purposeful, and relatively stable behaviors that can be described or explained. The concept of *pattern* relates to all parts of the system as well as to the relationship between the parts.

2. The behavioral system has many tasks to perform in order to maintain its integrity, which it does through the integration and effectiveness of its organized parts. Complex systems that are highly organized have more parts or subsystems.

    The recognition of these parts/subsystems (also supportive of Chin) gives greater clarity to this system, so it provides a foundation for more specifics for nursing practice. The seven subsystems identified are: attachment/affiliation, dependency, ingestion, elimination, sexuality, aggression, and achievement.

3. Each subsystem has drives or goals, a predisposition to act, a scope of possible actions, and behavioral actions.

These four elements within each subsystem assist in explaining a particular behavior. Thus, a particular system such as achievement might be modeled as shown in Figure 6-5.

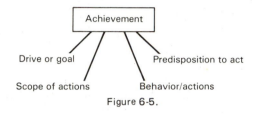

Figure 6-5.

4. Nursing problems stem from a problem within the system reflecting behavior that is less than optimal.

Thus, nursing is viewed as facilitating the behavioral system by supporting its balance through restoration and maintenance activities.

Models

From this theory emerges a behavioral systems model reflective of Chin's approach seen in Figure 6-6.

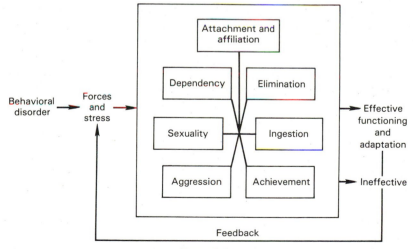

Figure 6-6.

The concepts in this behavioral system are abstract, inferential, and rather empirical. They are also reflective of a view of humans from a somewhat biological, psychological, and sociological framework. As usual, the more biological the concept, the more empirical it is, and the more psychological, the more abstract; the range is shown in Figure 6-7.

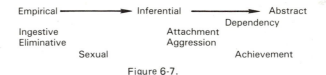

Figure 6-7.

Scale of Abstractions of Concepts/Subsystems

Johnson offers no clear group of characteristics (or concepts) of these subsystems, but she does attempt to explain the difficulty or error in viewing them narrowly within a systems theory. For example, the sexual subsystem not only is biological but also is part of the role, procreation, and gratification behavior related to marriage, such as courting and mating, which strongly relate to sexuality. Thus certain characteristics of each concept can be thought of as empirical (such as frequency and duration), while others are more inferential (such as certain mating behaviors). Although ingestion is basically biological, one's appetite, or why and how much one eats, can be harder to measure, so the concept becomes inferential. The placement of these subsystems on the scale is truly arbitrary, depending on one's way of thinking and on what specific characteristics one would identify for each. Thus the approach to patient care based on these parts/subsystems will vary depending on how the nurse defines each one, unless specific characteristics are universally developed for each through investigation and research. As with need-oriented theories, the clarity of needs/concepts is greater when they are biologically/empirically oriented than when they are psychologically oriented.

Although systems theory emphasizes the whole and breaks down the interacting parts more for discussion than for reality, there is within most of the nursing theories a rather segmented view. Although the subsystems truly interact and almost blend when one tries to develop characteristics, some are basically biological (ingestion and elimination), some psychological (dependency and aggression), and others somewhat psychosocial in nature (achievement and attachment).

Application to Nursing Process

The focus of the nursing process (as noted in Table 6-3) is on the behaviors of individuals, who represent a total system with parts or subsystems. The amount of assessment data that one can gather from a particular patient is, from a holistic framework, enormous. It is, therefore, essential to focus on a particular stress or force that is affecting certain subsystems, even though every force affects the total system and thus every subsystem. For example, a patient who has suddenly lost a spouse has a major disruption within the attachment subsystem. Behaviors that will affect their dependency, ingestion, and achievement will no doubt also be affected. The nurse will identify those behaviors that affect the system most and establish priorities before implementating care. One who has difficulty eating needs more immediate attention in relation to the ingestion subsystem than in relation to the dependency subsystem. In other words, the nurse looks at the individual's total behavior in relation to stress and decides which subsystems need attention at the moment. This should *not* be interpreted in so narrow a context as to support a nursing approach oriented toward a very specific area or behavior. A nurse who provides water at a patient's request without assessing its impact on elimination, dependency, and attachment behavior is not approaching nursing from Johnson's theoretical framework.

In using the nursing process with the subsystem, it is important to remember the four elements mentioned within the theory. When assessing the individual's interpersonal shells (subsystem affiliation), the nurse needs to identify both the goals for the interaction and the scope of possibilities in terms of relating to others, and then predict the position and pattern of relating and identify the reason for the choice of a particular behavior. Just knowing the individual's interpersonal behaviors is not adequate. This type of assessment takes a great deal of time, but without it, little or no effective nursing can occur—a reminder that without theory, no process is effective.

Evaluation

Johnson's theory incorporates Chin's systems approach to nursing. Their approaches to the general concepts of systems theory are identical. The parts/subsystems are identified with little real explana-

Table 6-3

Nursing Process and Johnson's Theory

Stages	Basic Approach	Nursing Approaches
Assessment	Information/data/observations Examine patient behavior in relation to each subsystem and the interactive behavior of the subsystem. Review the scope of possible actions/behaviors, the driving force, the predisposition to act (patterns), and reasons for the specific behavior.	Implications for gathering data Obtain assessment data that is relevant to some force or stress within the individual's life that is affecting his behavior. *Subsystem* *Data* (examples only) Attachment/affiliation What are the patient's interpersonal skills? What support systems are available? Elimination What behaviors are manifested in the excretion of waste? Ingestion What are the eating habits? Dependency How does the patient respond to nurturance and assistance? Aggression How does the individual protect himself from stresses? Sexuality What is the attitude toward procreation? Achievement What are the career goals, and what behaviors support these goals? *Subsystem Interaction Data* (examples) How is the individual's aggressive behavior affecting his attachment and dependency behaviors? Is the lack of proper food influencing the elimination pattern? Is the individual's sex role identification influencing career achievements?

	Information/data/observations	Implications for gathering data
Diagnosis	Identify the problems/stress affecting the system as a whole, a subsystem, or some subsystems; it reflects some type of behavioral difficulty that is hindering an effectively functioning system.	Diagnostic categories can relate to: 1. The system as a whole, e.g., environmental stress causing ineffective behavior to support a holistically functioning individual. 2. Each subsystem or interaction between subsystems, such as inability to achieve on the job due to poor interpersonal/affiliative behaviors.
Plan	Identify actions that will facilitate behavior that supports the system and inhibit those that do not.	Behaviors need to be reinforced when they support the system as a whole, such as communicating existing patterns or goals on the part of the patient. Behaviors that are characteristic of a subsystem, such as reducing the patient's dependence by teaching him to care for himself.
Implementation	Utilize those behaviors that facilitate effective functioning.	Nursing behaviors that provide for each subsystem. For example, the nurse monitors intake (ingestion) that will facilitate the elimination of wastes. The interaction between the nurse and patient facilitates independence.
Evaluation	Reassess in terms of output behaviors that have provided adaptation and effective functioning of the total behavioral system.	Gather additional information about those subsystems that were particularly affected by forces or stress and identify their impact on other subsystems.

tion of their characteristics, which makes it very difficult to utilize this theory in nursing practice. Many questions arise as to where certain human behaviors fit within the subsystems. Some behaviors that are not included in the broad category are fairly obvious. For example, one can assume that within the subsystem of ingestion is the intake of air and the sense of smell. But are affiliative behaviors, such as having a close relationship, also under the sexuality subsystem? It is difficult to separate, at least for assessment, whether dominant or passive behavior relates more to the achievement or to the aggression subsystem. Perhaps these differences or the categorizations of such behaviors are not important, as long as we consistently relate to the whole.

The theory is relatively easy to understand if one is familiar with general systems theory. The concepts within the model do not contradict the theoretical approach, and the assumptions are sound. As a theory it does provide an explanation for and a way of describing human behavior. It does not predict outcomes except to say that if the behaviors are effective, the system will adapt to stressors. Nursing deals with individuals when they are experiencing crisis or illness, which are forms of stress.

MARTHA ROGERS: DESCRIPTION OF THE THEORY

Rogers believes that the uniqueness of nursing relates to its focus, which is *unitary man* within an open system. The science of nursing is the study of unitary man and seeks to develop knowledge that describes, explains, and predicts for nursing practice. Thus Rogers supports the development and use of theory as primary for the nursing profession.

The emphasis of this theory is *man/environment*, which is indivisible using the systems approach. The concepts of health and nursing are less significant and are generally explained in reference to the two major concepts. Rogers believes that it is only through the knowledge of man/environment and their interaction that nursing can truly understand clients and assist them to achieve health, which is the purpose of nursing.

Certain assumptions are basic to Rogers's theoretical framework, as noted in Table 6-4. All of these assumptions are supportive of systems theory, for example, those related to holism, differentiation, and order. Rogers's notion that man/environment is inseparable truly supports the open systems ideology. Approaching human be-

Table 6-4

Rogers's Assumptions of Man/Environment

Assumption	Related Concepts and Definition of Terms	Significance
Mankind has integrity and characteristics that reflect a unified whole.	Holism—viewing living organisms as interacting wholes rather than as the sum of their parts	Viewing individuals from a biopsychosocial framework is inappropriate.
	Integrity—state of completeness	
Mankind/environment constantly exchanges matter and energy.	Entropy—supports degradation and disorder of matter and energy and the lack of organization within the system (not open-system oriented)	Supports open systems theory. Supports negentropy rather than entropy which, for example, views aging as a creative process rather than a running-down process. An energy field is a totally unifying concept in terms of the universe and how we should view it.
	Negentropy—increasing order of complexity and heterogeneity (dissimilarity)	
	Energy field—basically an electrically charged field which is infinite and is the fundamental unit of all living and nonliving things	
Life processes are evolutionary, which is irreversible and unidirectional within a space and time continuum.	Evolution—process by which the whole universe is in progression with its interrelated events	Supports the idea of negentropy since human beings are becoming more complex all the time. The speed of change varies with the different age groups. The whole developmental continuum becomes more unidirectional and more complex.
	Continuum—characteristic of something that is continuous and in which a fundamental common character is discernible amid a series of insensible or indefinite variations.	
Mankind's wholeness within the energy field has rhythm, pattern, and organization.	Rhythm—ordered recurrent alternation of strong and weak elements	Rhythm does exist holistically, as in sleep and wake patterns. Humans have a self-regulating ability to maintain themselves while experiencing change. Thus, understanding their patterns of behavior in relation to change gives us strong clues to understanding human characteristics.
	Pattern—involves a sample of traits, acts, or other observable features that are in continuous change so that new patterns emerge	
	Organization—arrangement of elements within a system into a whole of interdependent parts	
Mankind's humanness is reflective of the capacity for abstraction, feelings, language, thought, sensation, and emotion.	Sentience—an awareness of feelings or reactions to stimulation	Humans, through their feelings and ability to think abstractly, are creative in their view and understanding of the world.

ings holistically within a framework of organization and sentience provides quite a different way of seeing patients/clients than via the need theories approach or the behavioral systems approach of Johnson.

Rogers would disagree with Chin and Johnson in terms of identifying the parts or subsystems. Rogers is consistent in her holistic approach and continues to identify what she calls *unifying concepts*. Note that the concepts identified in Table 6-4 do *not* reflect any biological, psychological, or sociological components or parts but rather are concepts such as *energy* and *pattern* that are related to *wholeness*. The concept of wholeness is also incorporated in relation to human behavior. Concepts such as objective, subjective, internal, and external are not appropriate for her within the reality of wholeness.

Rogers provides certain principles of nursing science called *homeodynamics*, which are viewed as life processes. The word *homeodynamics* is used in contrast to the concept *homeostasis*. *Homeo*- means similar or like, -*stasis* focuses on relative stability between different but independent elements within a system, and -*dynamic* reflects a state of change and growth of an object or event. Thus *homeodynamics* are consistent with systems theory and *homeostasis* is not. The three principles of this life process are helicy, resonancy, and integrality.

Helicy. Helicy involves human/environment rhythmic interaction within an evolutionary negentropic process within space and time.

Helic- is derived from Greek and means *spiral*. Thus helicy connotes evolution within an open system as innovative change increasing and moving within a period of time or space. Note the spiral model shown in Figure 6-8; view the line in the center as evolutionary change, the change/evolution spiral itself as supporting patterns, and the whole model with an open environment. Helicy supports all the assumptions and their concepts as stated previously. Thus, the spiral in the model reflects movement that has pattern, organization, rhythm, integrity, and holism, and is goal directed. The spiral has all these characteristics. Also included are reciprocy (mutual exchange) and synchrony (recurring coexistence) which reflect the man/environment relationship within the spiral. Another way of characterizing helicy is to say that humans and environment are exchanging energy forces and coexisting within an evolutionary process.

Resonancy. Resonancy is characteristic of the changes within the human/enviornment (energy field) and involves the intensifica-

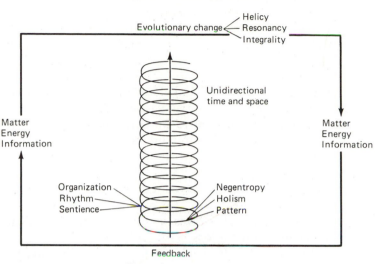

Figure 6-8. Spiral model.

tion, enrichment, and vibration that are reflective of lower or higher wave patterns.

This principle gives a greater dimension to evolutionary change. It not only is continuous but also varies in degree of intensity at different times.

Integrality. Integrality (previously called *complementarity*) is the continuous process of uniting or blending the human field and the environment into an integrated whole.

This reinforces the holistic concept of humans and the view that humans cannot be separated from the total environment because they are an energy field within the environment.

These three principles are useful in nursing because they assist us in understanding humans, the environment, and change. Within this frame of reference, aging becomes part of a natural evolutionary process with the following characteristics:

helicy—Change is innovative, moving along with a spiral pattern.

resonancy—Change varies with intensity at different times.

integrality—Changes occur within the context of the individual as part of the environment.

Thus, in looking at rest and sleep patterns or taste pattern, we know that they change in intensity with age in a unique, innovative way as influenced by the environment.

The following statements or assumptions which can be drawn from the model may be of assistance in clarifying a theory which is very abstract:

1. If one studies an individual's *pattern* of behavior over a period of time, certain characteristics will emerge that are in some way both common to humans and unique to the individual. For example, if someone loses a loved one, it is essential to obtain a historical perspective on how the individual has previously coped with loss, with the goal of reinforcing positive and successful behaviors. (As noted in the spiral, the pattern repeats itself over and over again with some change). Such information also gives us clues about how all humans tend to handle such a loss.

2. Since humans and the environment (integrality) are basically inseparable, it is more appropriate to gather information relating to the interaction between them. Focusing on understanding humans first and then the environment would not be as helpful, since it is their integration that explains the world event. If individuals were to become less than healthy, and we assessed first their condition and then the environment for pollution without identifying their relationship or "oneness as a force," we would not achieve a change toward health. Another way of viewing this is to focus on a health-oriented human/environment rather than on health in relation to humans and health in relation to environment.

3. Humans/environment experience different degrees and intensities (resonancy) of change (evolution). Changes in technology and within the health field are occurring at a much faster pace than they had previously. Such changes increase the energy and information flow, requiring a greater degree of organization. This pace affects the energy field, the human/ environment interaction. Thus, individuals who experience additional changes, such as a reduced health state, may have a reduced ability to expend additional energy. For example, if a single parent who is the sole support of herself and her children becomes unemployed, it is possible that the amount of energy she needs in order to deal with the change may be unavailable. In such a case, she may behave in less acceptable ways, such as abusing the children, which actually creates more, instead of fewer, difficulties. The focus of support for

this woman would be to assist her in such a way that she can increase energy and can pattern her behavior in more successful ways.

Application to the Nursing Process

The nursing process is utilized to help the nurse to focus on the human being's holistic pattern. As noted in Table 6-5, the assumptions and homeodynamic process provide a frame of reference in which increasing change is the focus. Compare Rogers's model (Figure 6-8) with the use of the nursing process (Table 6-5). The assessment focuses on the input—energy—and the output—evaluation, or the changes in the use of that changing energy. The diagnosis, plan, and implementation deal with the individual's feelings or sentience, pattern, holism, and so on, noted in the center of the model. As with the nursing process, the model, with its spiral and its feedback system, especially during evaluation, continuously repeats itself somewhat differently with each repetition.

The following clinical situation is an example of how the assumptions and principles can be incorporated:

CLINICAL SITUATION

Ms. Sullivan, who is a thirty-year-old married woman, enters the prenatal clinic with her five-year-old daughter. Ms. Sullivan is requesting an examination because she believes that she is three months pregnant. She offers no complaints and feels relatively healthy.

Assessment Data	Assumptions/Principles
What is Ms. Sullivan's interaction with the health personnel and with her five-year-old daughter within the clinic environment?	Integrality (Human/environment integrated)
What was her previous maternity experience like?	Patterns, organization of previous evolutionary changes.
	Resonancy—degree and intensity of experience.
How does she feel about the pregnancy?	Negentropy—increasing complexity
	Sentience—feelings and reactions
What changes has she experienced in the last three months?	Helicy—evolutionary changes

The assessment data listed will lead the nurse to care for Ms. Sullivan in a way that is reflective of Rogers's theory. Note the direction

Table 6-5

Nursing Process and Rogers's Theory

Stages	Basic Approach	Nursing Approaches
Assessment	Focus on human-environment interaction, energy pattern, and organization within the context of the degree of change.	Gather data about the individual's previous ways of interacting with the environment. Identify the degree of change that the individual is experiencing. Study patterns of behavior in terms of the use of energy to achieve health. *Example*—With a newly hospitalized patient, identify ways in which the environment interacts with the patient in terms of the use of energy. Does the hospital routine facilitate the patient's rest patterns? Does the individual have the energy to handle pain and reduced mobility?
Diagnosis	Identify certain patterns in relation to the human/environment interaction.	Diagnostic categories are reflective of a particular pattern of behaving. *Example*—Inability to deal with body image changes.
Plan	Identify actions that support the achievement of health and welfare.	Plan to support positive patterns of behavior. *Example*—Provide ways of increasing the person's ability to respond to changes in ability to ambulate.
Implementation	Support behaviors oriented toward improving the individual's ability to handle change.	Support patient during ambulation and reinforce previous positive behaviors. Provide activities that reinforce a positive self-image. *Example*—Assist individual to walk as he previously did while focusing on available energy.
Evaluation	Reassess behavioral patterns and the interaction between human/environment in relation to health and welfare.	Continue to review the level of energy available to handle changes and to respond in a more mature manner.

the nurse's thinking will *not* take—it will not be disease oriented, skill oriented, or need focused. Pregnancy is viewed as a developmental human experience, and the nurse's role is to facilitate the evolutionary change by understanding the change in matter, energy, and information.

Evaluation

Rogers's theory is one of the most abstract nursing theories and requires the understanding of a set of terms that are mostly unfamiliar. The view of *human/environment* is very broad and may appear difficult to use in a nursing situation. Going from an empirical, largely biological framework to Rogers's theory may appear like one giant step, but the theory explains the human condition with a greater sense of reality because it provides a way of viewing change. Many questions arise that need to be answered through research in order to better incorporate the theory into practice. For example, what patterns are most functional within healthy individuals? What intensity (resonancy) of change is appropriate at different age levels? To what degree does the human capacity for sentience (creativity and feelings) support or interfere with one's life capabilities? During a period of low energy input, what is the approximate level of change and how are patterns affected?

Rogers's theory is quite complex, unless one has a strong scientific background, especially in physics. It attempts to describe and explain the universe and, if used correctly, could assist one in predicting outcomes through a careful understanding of patterns that are repetitive and similar. The theory supports Ludwig von Bertalanffy's in its definitions and approaches, while clarifying somewhat the ways in which open-system theory can be incorporated into nursing practice.

What is significantly different about Rogers's model is the lack of subsystems, or parts within the core; instead there is a frame of reference that continues to support holism. Since Rogers did not specifically provide a model, the one shown in Figure 6-8 is interpretive and based on her stated assumptions. Had she provided a model, one could have examined the relationship between the model and the assumptions to see if there were any contradictions. The concepts are abstract, and even with her definitions, clarity is not reached. Many of the terms are unfamiliar for the most part, and it is difficult to develop specific clarifying characteristics. Concepts such as holism, rhythm, and helicy do not provide an easy explanation for health or stress. It is inappropriate to make deductions that make humans an assortment of parts to explain their physical or emotional behavior. The concepts explain the nature of the environment of which humans are a part in a very encompassing manner. We are so empirically oriented in our everyday lives that it takes real effort to take a holistic world view.

IMOGENE KING: DESCRIPTION OF THE THEORY

King's theory builds on von Bertalanaffy's, focusing on *human beings* interacting with the *environment.* The basic assumption is that *nursing* involves caring for human beings, with the goal of *health* Health involves adjustments to stressors in the internal and external environment. The four basic concepts of nursing theories (in italics) are significant to the theory.

The framework includes three interacting systems—personal, interpersonal, and social. The interactions, which are basically reflective of the interpersonal system of nurse/client, include perception, judgment, reaction, and transaction on the parts of both nurse and client. The concepts noted under each interacting system are shown below. The interpersonal system is most emphasized within the theory.

Personal	*Interpersonal*	*Social*
Perception	Interaction	Organization
Self	Communication	Authority
Growth and development	Transaction	Power
Body image	Role	Status
Space	Stress	Decision making
Time		

These sixteen concepts and their interrelationship represent the basis of the theory. The following definitions of characteristics of the concepts are provided by King in *A Theory of Nursing.*

Personal

> *Perception*—the individual's representation of reality, which is universal, subjective, active-oriented, and involves organizing, interpreting, and transforming information (pp. 20-23)

> *Self*—characteristic of a dynamic individual within an open system who is goal oriented; reflects the sum total (ideas, attitudes, and values) of who one is (pp. 26-27).

Growth and development—continuous change of patterns based on one's endowment, experiences, and environment (pp. 30–31)

Body image—one's perception of one's own body and others' reactions to one's appearance

Space—the physical area existing in all directions having characteristics that are universal, personal, and situational (pp. 36–37)

Time—the duration between two events; it is irreversible, relational, durational, measurable, and subjective.

These concepts closely relate to one another. Our growth and development have a strong impact on our perception of body image, time, and space. Our perception of space can have a strong impact on our perception of time; time seems to pass slowly, for example, when we are in a crowded elevator. Perception can also influence our growth and development, especially if we have negative experiences. These concepts represent King's description of human beings. They are supportive of an open-systems approach, recognizing humans as having patterns, and changing and interacting with the environment. The concept of *holism* is more strongly supported than behavior theory is, since personal systems are not divided up into parts, as they are according to Johnson.

Interpersonal

Interaction—verbal and nonverbal behavior between two or more individuals

Communication—the interchange of thoughts and opinions among individuals; can be either verbal or nonverbal

Transaction—the transfer of value between two or more persons which is unique and based on experience and goal-directed behaviors

Role—a set of expected behaviors with rules that define rights and obligations that affect the interaction between two or more persons

Stress—negative or positive energy response of the individual to persons, objects, and events called stressors

The definitions of the concepts related to interpersonal systems reinforce the concepts noted in the category of personal systems. Interaction is based on one's perception of space and time. Communication and stress are affected by one's stage of growth and development as well as by one's perceptions. The interpersonal concepts also strongly interrelate. Interactions are influenced by the way one communicates, how one sees one's role, the goals one has (transactions), and the environmental internal stress one feels.

Social

Organizational—social units having structure, functions, and resources to achieve goals

Authority—situation in which an individual accepts another's control in decision making

Power—a situational, dynamic, and goal-directed process that occurs when one or more persons can influence others

Status—the position of an individual or group within a social stratification; reversible and situational

Decision making—a continuous, goal-directed process used to reach a goal

The concepts noted within a social system are, in effect, the environmental forces that have an impact on the personal and interpersonal systems. They represent the forces within the external environment that give structure to organizations, such as hospitals or clinics, in which the nurse-patient interaction occurs. The concepts as defined by King can, for the most part, be understood by inference or are abstract. For example, the concept *power,* which can be understood mostly by observation (for example, by inference) is described in terms of a particular changing situation as related to a goal. King further describes *power* as having energy, as needed to enhance group wholesomeness related to authority, and as a function of human interactions and decision making. The concept *body image* is probably more abstract than *power,* because it is not seen in reference to a particular situation, but instead occurs within a person. *Body image* is what one thinks about one's body and how one feels others react to one's appearance. Another abstract concept is *interpersonal.* It is not a particular theory but an action going on between individuals. The question of whether these concepts are more or less abstract or of whether one can really characterize them as inferential, because they can be described by observation, is a difficult one. Research during an interpersonal exchange is necessary in order to better understand their meaning. Using King's definitions facilitates a clearer understanding of the concepts within the theory.

Model

The model shown in Figure 6-9 incorporates all the basic concepts in King's theory of goal attainment. It is both circular and linear, because it has a core (interpersonal) and the components have

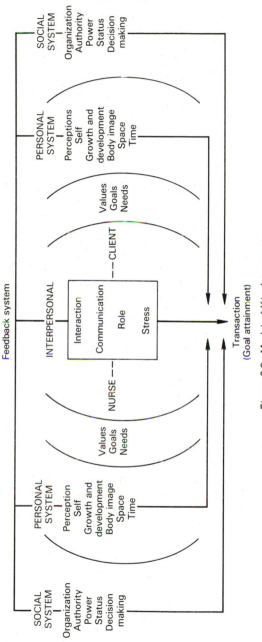

Figure 6-9. Model of King's concepts.

a direction. It reflects an open-systems approach to the interactive process occurring between the nurse and the client. At the core is the nurse-client interaction, which occurs through verbal and nonverbal communication based on their identified roles and the perceived stress. Both the nurse and the client have a personal and a social system affecting that interaction. For example, the client's perception of his status and of the nurse's status can strongly influence whether a particular goal is achieved.

King offers certain propositions that are supported by the model developed in this book. For example, if transactions are made during the nurse-client interaction, growth and development will be enhanced. Note the feedback system, which leads to transaction. Review the following propositions and see if they are valid utilizing the model presented in Figure 6-9.

1. Both the nurse's and the client's values are influenced by their perceptions of themselves and their status.
2. The verbal and nonverbal communications that occur between the nurse and the client are affected by their perceptions of time and space, and by the authority that each perceives the other has.
3. Mutual decision making within the context of the nurse's and client's perception of their needs influences goal attainment.
4. The perceived level of stress on the part of both the nurse and the client is influenced by their perceptions of themselves and by the organization in which they find themselves.

All these propositions are valid and contain concepts within each system of the theory. For example, the first proposition identifies the concepts *nurse* and *client* (interpersonal), the concept *perception* (personal system), and the concept *status* (social system). Thus, using the model and relating the identified concepts provides for the development of valid propositions (assumptions) which can be tested through research and, if validated, used for nursing practice.

Application to Nursing Process

King supports the Goal-Oriented Nursing Record (GONR) approach to the nursing process (see Table 6-6). The terminology differs somewhat but the process is similar. Each step needs to be viewed from the framework of each part of King's system as well as in an integrated manner.

Table 6-6

Nursing Process and King's Theory

Nursing Process (King's Goal-Oriented Nursing Record/GONR)	Personal System	Interpersonal System	Social System
	Data Gathered		
Assessment through communication	Nurse's and client's perceptions of who they are	Nurse's and client's abilities to communicate in relation to each's role	Decision-making abilities of the client and nurse
Interaction (gather subjective and objective data)	Level of growth and development; Perception of body image, time, and space	Level of stress; Individual's ability to function in his usual role	The status and power afforded the nurse by the client
	Problem-Oriented		
Diagnosis (monitor problems and/or changes as negative or positive)	Ability to enhance one's growth and development or accept one's body image	Ability to deal with stress and to communicate	Client's ability to accept or reject authority and make appropriate decisions

Table 6-6 (cont.)

Nursing Process (King's Goal-Oriented Nursing Record/GONR)	Personal System	Interpersonal System	Social System
		Identify Ways to Resolve Problems	
Plan (means agreed upon to resolve the problem and attain the goal)	Identify mutual goals and the needed action of nurse and client in relation to values and needs of each and in relation to the client's body image	Validate nurse's and client's perceptions of space and time in order to improve communication and reduce stress	Utilize power and authority of nurse to educate client
Implementation (action to resolve problem)	Support behaviors that enhance an understanding of self and growth and development	Communicate and facilitate the client's goal by reducing stress	Allow client to make decisions regarding care after teaching
		Gather Further Data	
Evaluate (assess outcome of goals)	Difference in perception of body image	Level of stress after communicating	Assess new level of knowledge

The assessment, which is the subjective and objective information, relates to such factors as the client's and nurse's perceptions and the client's ability to communicate and make decisions. For example, a ten-year-old client who was in a car accident and cannot move his arm will subjectively complain of pain. The swelling around his elbow is the objective data. Additional information/date can be gathered on the effect of this injury on his growth, development, and activities, and on his body image now that his elbow is broken. His perception of the time and place of the accident may influence his behavior. If the accident occurred very late at night in an area of which his parents disapproved, additional stress will be evident and will affect his ability to communicate.

The problem/diagnosis will relate to the degree of pain he is experiencing and to whether he can function adequately without help in meeting his personal needs. The plan would call for reducing his pain and supporting his elbow to enhance appropriate growth and development of his bones. The nurse would also plan to teach this client ways of supporting his arm to reduce later swelling. The mutual goal is to reduce pain, and that can be achieved.

The major focus of this theory is goal attainment. Thus, whatever the data, diagnosis, or plan, the critical test of the success of utilizing this theory is whether a mutually agreed upon goal had been achieved. This is viewed within the framework of the client's and nurse's perceptions of the world. Simply stated, the theory involves two individuals within a social system interacting with each other based on their perception of the world in order to achieve a client-centered goal, within the framework of a client problem.

Evaluation

King approaches her theory from a theoretical framework. Her theory of goal attainment (as she calls it) offers defined concepts and a limited model which emphasizes that individuals' perceptions influence their reactions and interactions in relation to their goals. Her propositions are supported by her definitions of the concepts. The terms used within the theory are not difficult to understand, as the reader is probably already familiar with most of them.

Although the theory characterizes *humans* as sentient, rational, social, reactive, perceptive, and purposeful in nature, which is a holistic framework, the orientation toward problems is likely to encourage the nurse to deal with the biological or psychological parts of the individual. This can lead to confusion and some difficulty in applying the theory to practice. The concept of *health* is discussed in terms of stress, the environment, and the achievement of one's maximum potential for daily living. The apparent relationship between *health* and *transaction* is in terms of the goal; thus, the goal must be health oriented. *Nursing* is viewed in relation to the nurse's perceptions of the client's problems, which are mostly based on the nurse's needs and values. The *environment* is reflective of her social system, which is somewhat limited.

The theory with its three interlocking systems is not clear. It is evident that King incorporates the nurse and the client into the interpersonal systems, and the concept *perception* within the personal system, but it is unclear whether both the client's and nurse's characteristics are included in the concepts related to the social system. The model assumes that all three systems relate to both the client and the nurse, but the theory does not make it completely clear that this is correct. This theory, like others relating to systems theory, does provide for *input*—the nurse/client interaction, *process*—the reactions and transactions, and *output*—the achievement of goals with a feedback system. This feedback system is supported by the constant interaction of the three systems. Also supportive of systems theory are the concepts and definitions related to time and space and human beings existing within an open system. The emphasis on organization and humans interacting within the environment with a purpose or goal is strongly reflective of systems theory.

King's theory is helpful in explaining and describing a client/nurse situation. At this point, it cannot predict outcome and goals for practice. In the final chapter of her book, King encourages research in recognition of this fact.

BETTY NEUMAN:
DESCRIPTION OF THE THEORY

Neuman describes her theory as the health care systems model, a total-person approach to patient problems. As Neuman states in *The Neuman Systems Model: Application to Nursing Education and Practice,* the purpose of this model is to explain the function of *nursing,* which is "to assist *individuals, families, and groups* to attain and maintain a maximum level of total *wellness* by purposeful interventions". The major concepts are stress and its reduction, and the individual's interactions within the *environment.* The four major concepts are well identified. The model is quite similar to Chin's in its emphasis on stress and strain as the input, the inner parts are representing the physiological, psychological, sociocultural, and developmental factors, and the output as reflecting a state of stress reduction. The feedback system is represented as reconstitution, whereby the information about the reduced level of stress is incorporated into the input system for further analysis.

Models

Neuman provides a model for her theory which can facilitate the development of assumptions/propositions. The model, shown in Figure 6-10, is basically linear and directional, with a core identification (see Chapter 2) that is central to the model. It shows multiple relationships among the various factors that influence the basic structure of the individual and his ability to deal with stress. Within each of the boxes there are identified relationships to the circle (core), whch are the characteristics of the concepts. It is the core of the circle that projects the meaning of the model. The boxes are peripheral and have an impact on the core and on each other.

Neuman made certain assumptions in the development of this model. The following are a few of the assumptions that can be suppoted within the model.

Assumption	*Area within the Model*
Individuals are unique, but they also have common "knowns" or characteristics.	Basic structures and energy resources are within the core. (Note the list of structures pointing to the center of the circle.)
Stressors have the potential to disturb the normal lines of defense or the individual's equilibrium.	Stressors are outside the core and are affected by the lines of defense and resistance.
Primary prevention relates to the identification of risk factors associated with stress.	The area of primary prevention includes the reduction of stressors (note the line going from *primary prevention* to *stressors,* which then lead to both the *flexible* and *normal lines of defense*) and the strengthening of the flexible line of defense.
Secondary prevention relates to the symptoms, interventions, and treatment needed during illness.	Under secondary prevention, early case finding and the treatment of symptoms relates to the reactions of stress (note the line and arrows from *reaction* to *secondary prevention*) and the degree of reaction (within the edge of the circle).
Tertiary prevention relates to the adaptive process and reconstitution.	Under tertiary prevention are included readaptation, reeducation, and maintenance of stability (note the lines and arrows between *tertiary prevention* and *reconstitution*).

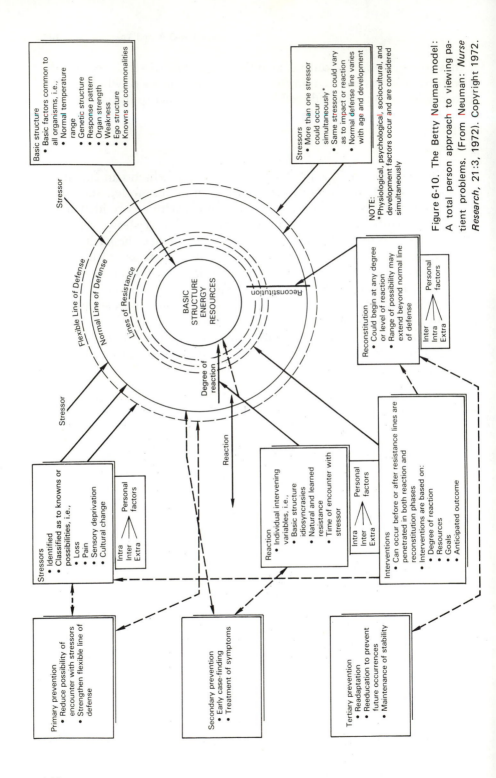

Figure 6-10. The Betty Neuman model: A total person approach to viewing patient problems. (From Neuman: *Nurse Research*, 21:3, 1972). Copyright 1972.

Basic structure
• Basic factors common to all organisms, i.e.,
   • Normal temperature range
   • Genetic structure
   • Response pattern
   • Organ strength
   • Weakness
   • Ego structure
   • Knowns or commonalities

Stressors
• More than one stressor could occur simultaneously*
• Same stressors could vary as to impact or reaction
• Normal defense line varies with age and development

NOTE:
*Physiological, psychological, sociocultural, and development factors occur and are considered simultaneously

Flexible Line of Defense
Normal Line of Defense
Lines of Resistance

Stressor

BASIC STRUCTURE ENERGY RESOURCES

Reconstitution

Reconstitution
• Could begin at any degree or level of reaction
• Range of possibility may extend beyond normal line of defense

Inter
Intra   Personal factors
Extra

Degree of reaction

Reaction

Stressor

Stressors
• Identified
• Classified as to knowns or possibilities, i.e.,
   • Loss
   • Pain
   • Sensory deprivation
   • Cultural change

Intra
Inter   Personal factors
Extra

Reaction
• Individual intervening variables, i.e.,
   • Basic structure idiosyncrasies
   • Natural and learned resistance
   • Time of encounter with stressor

Intra
Inter   Personal factors
Extra

Interventions
• Can occur before or after resistance lines are penetrated in both reaction and reconstitution phases
• Interventions are based on:
   • Degree of reaction
   • Resources
   • Goals
   • Anticipated outcome

Primary prevention
• Reduce possibility of encounter with stressors
• Strengthen flexible line of defense

Secondary prevention
• Early case-finding
• Treatment of symptoms

Tertiary prevention
• Readaptation
• Reeducation to prevent future occurrences
• Maintenance of stability

Other more specific and more graphic relationships can be identified within the model. Review the model (Fig. 6-10) and follow these assumptions.

One's genetic structure affects one's energy resources. (Note under *basic structure* the *genetic structure* and the arrow going from the box labeled *basic structure* to the inner circle related to *energy.*)

Assumption	Area within the Model
Stressors are *intrapersonal*—emerging from within the individual, *interpersonal*—occurring between two or more individuals, and *extrapersonal*—outside the individual.	There are two areas in which the model identifies these factors. One is just below the *stressors,* which explains where the stressors emerge. The other is below *reconstitution,* which explains that after intervention the stressors emerge differently in relation to their degree or to the individual's line of defense.

Early case finding can affect the degree of the reaction to a stressor. (Note *case finding* under *secondary prevention,* then follow the dotted arrows to the circle and the *degree of reaction.* In this case *secondary prevention* relates to *reaction,* which also relates to the *degree of reaction.*

In a way, all the items in the model affect the *basic structure energy resources.* All areas have arrows to the circle, except that there are indirect relationships noted between *primary, secondary,* and *tertiary prevention* and the circle. This theory provides a frame of reference or a way of looking at the health care system and the patient that is quite inclusive.

Although the model basically focuses on an individual, it is equally appropriate to view its usefulness in terms of the family or a community. Families have a basic structure and an energy level as well as the ability to deal with outside stressors in terms of their idiosyncrasies and previously learned behavior. Nurses intervene with individuals and families based on their goals, resources, and anticipated outcomes.

The most significant concept, which is well represented in the model, is *stress* and the individual's reaction to it within the environment. This supports the open-systems approach. Neuman uses Selye's definition of *stress* as tension-producing stimuli that can cause disequilibrium and crisis. Thus, that which Neuman calls *stress,* and Johnson calls *behavioral disorder* or *forces* and stress, and Rogers calls *energy,* and Roy, as you will see later, calls *stimuli,* are very similar in that they are all input factors. According to Webster's dictionary, *stress* means strain, pressure, and force. The concept *stress* is basically abstract and should be viewed as having a neutral state, because stress can be either positive or negative depending on the individual's reaction to it. The degree of stress is also difficult to explain: Some persons may be perceived as being under a great deal of stress when they do not exhibit symptoms; others may have few identifiable signs of stress but may experience many internal symptoms. An individual's line of defense or ability to resist stress is quite abstract in nature. We can only see the results when there is a weak line of resistance to disease; we are unable to truly monitor a strong or normal line of defense except to assume it is present if we are well.

Using Chin's approach to systems theory, and eliminating some of the specific criteria noted within Neuman's model, a different model (Fig. 6-11) could emerge.

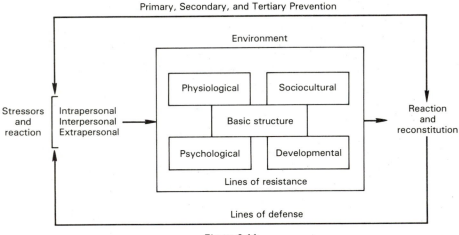

Figure 6-11.

Within this model the major concepts and their relationships are identified and the assumptions supported. Some of the criteria that Neuman identifies under each of the concepts are incomplete; the model need not include them. For example, the criteria under *basic structure* in Neuman's model identify seven basic factors related to temperature, genetic structure, response pattern, and so on. Some are more empirical and inferential, such as *temperature* and *organ strength* (heart strength), while others are quite abstract, such as *ego structure* and *response pattern.* The last one, *knowns* or *commonalities,* is too vague a concept to classify and probably represents all other factors not noted.

Other concepts relating to basic structures could be identified, such as energy level and blood pressure. It is possible that energy relates to *weakness* or *response pattern* and that blood pressure relates to *genetic structures* and *organ strength*. In looking at the concept *stressors,* those noted as examples in the model are *loss, pain,* and so on. Both *loss* and *pain* are abstract and require specific characteristics to clarify them for practice. Under this concept, one could develop an endless list of stressors that can be identified within an individual and within the environment.

Application to Nursing Process

Neuman provides three basic principles to consider when assessing an individual from the framework of her model:

1. All factors influencing a person's perceptual field are to be known.
2. The nurse must validate what the stressors mean to the patient.
3. The nurse's perception will influence her assessment of the patient's situation.

These all support King's emphasis on understanding the impact of the perceptions of the patient and nurse on the data that will be collected. Note that the model's main focus is on the characteristics of humans and their relationship to stress. The major areas to consider that relate to the use of the nursing process within the model are stress; perception; primary, secondary, and tertiary preventions; and the physiological, psychological, sociocultural, and developmental factors.

Within Table 6-7, the main areas need to be identified in such a way that they are all integrated at any given time. For example, in dealing with a patient who smokes, and who has been found by the physician to have no respiratory disease, but who is having a coughing reaction to the irritation caused by smoking, the nurse should focus on the following based on the assumption that smoking is a stress within the context of the physiological, psychological, sociocultural, and developmental factors:

Assessment—Assess the risk that smoking poses to normal lines of defense (primary prevention). Note the degree to which smoking affects the cough (secondary prevention). Assess the potential risk of the hazard (tertiary prevention).

Table 6-7

Nursing Process and Neuman's Model

Nursing Process	Primary Prevention (Risk Factor)	Secondary Prevention (Symptoms, Intervention, and Treatment)	Tertiary (Adaptive Process)
Assessment—gather data related to stressors within the context of the intrapersonal, interpersonal, and extrapersonal forces.	Identify potential risk or hazards of stressors to the normal lines of defense or resistance from a physiological, psychological, sociocultural, or developmental viewpoint based on the perceptions of the patient and the nurse.	Identify the degree of reaction to the stressor as related to the available resources and the nurse/patient perceptions of the symptoms that are evident (physiological, psychological, sociocultural, and developmental).	Note the patient's ability to adapt to the potential or real risks or hazards and maintain stability. Assess the need for reeducation
Diagnosis—reflects stressors or lines of defense and resistance.	Orient toward specific risks or hazards and the patient's ability to use his lines of defense and resistance.	Reflects symptoms/reactions to stressors.	Relates to specific needs for education or resources.
Plan—organize to reduce stressors or build defenses.	Identify actions that would reduce risks or hazards that have been diagnosed.	Organize those activities that will reduce the impact of the stressors, especially in relation to the physiological, psychological, sociocultural, and developmental factors.	Identify those behaviors that facilitate stability and cultural adaptation.
Implementation—activate behaviors that reduce stressors and build up lines of defense.	Provide education and reinforce behaviors.	Support patient in these attempts to cope with stresses; reduce maladaptive behavior by meeting patient's needs.	Reeducate and motivate patient.
Evaluation—assess outcome of reduction of stressors.		Reassess status of needs and the patient's ability to cope with stress.	Identify further need for education and behavior changes that facilitate adaptation.

Diagnosis—Reflects the patient's ability to handle smoking (primary), the symptoms manifested (secondary), and the specific needs in relation to motivation or education (tertiary).

Plan—Identify the patient/nurse behaviors that will enhance the patient's ability to resist the stressor (primary), reduce the symptoms caused by the stressor (secondary), and remotivate the patient to either stop or reduce his exposure to the stressor (tertiary).

Implementation—Follow the behaviors indicated by the plan, such as supporting a nonsmoking regime (primary); providing breathing exercises, medication, or behavior modification activities to reduce smoking and coughing (secondary); and continuing to support realistic goals to reduce the stressor of smoking (tertiary).

Evaluation—Reassess flexible and normal lines of defense in relation to smoking and the patient's cough (primary), monitor the cough (secondary), and remotivate and reeducate (tertiary).

If one continues to incorporate all the factors identified into an organized approach in which to view Neuman's theory and the nursing process in the area of assessment only, it might appear like Table 6-8.

From Table 6-8, it is evident that the theory can involve gathering an enormous amount of data/information. Thus it is essential to initially focus on a particular stressor in relation to specific factors, because it would be impossible and prohibitively time consuming to gather everything during the initial contact with the patient. One possibility in the case of the example described previously would be to primarily identify smoke as the stressor in relation to the intrapersonal, psychogenic, and physiologic response from the perspective of secondary prevention. Later the focus could shift to the interpersonal and sociocultural forces influencing the patient's ability to deal with the stressor. If the patient is an adolescent, the focus might shift to the developmental factors that make it difficult to reeducate or motivate the patient to reduce his exposure to the stressor (smoking).

Evaluation

Neuman's theory is truly a systems-model approach within the framework of stress. Her emphasis is on the individual and the environment as seen from an open-system approach. It supports the in-

Table 6-8

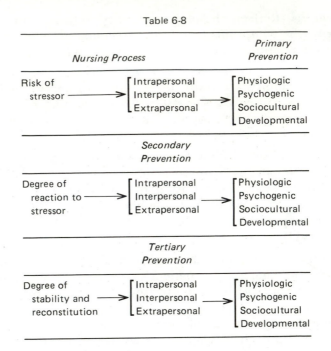

	Nursing Process	Primary Prevention
Risk of stressor ⟶	Intrapersonal Interpersonal Extrapersonal ⟶	Physiologic Psychogenic Sociocultural Developmental

	Secondary Prevention	
Degree of reaction to ⟶ stressor	Intrapersonal Interpersonal ⟶ Extrapersonal	Physiologic Psychogenic Sociocultural Developmental

	Tertiary Prevention	
Degree of stability and ⟶ reconstitution	Intrapersonal Interpersonal ⟶ Extrapersonal	Physiologic Psychogenic Sociocultural Developmental

terdependence and integration of the physiological, psychological, sociocultural, and developmental factors, which is consistent with Chin's model. The specific variables needed to identify those factors within the individual or the environment, and the details of how to integrate them are not offered. This leaves the theory open to many interpretations, which might be helpful at this stage of theory development. The theory is somewhat complicated in its presentation, and because there are so many abstract concepts noted within the model, it would, in totality, be difficult to incorporate into practice. In using it consistently for practice, priorities and critical judgments would be essential as well as time consuming.

The theory does provide a clear frame of reference with which to view a nursing situation that differs somewhat from other nursing theories. The major difference is the emphasis on stress and prevention. The theory can describe and explain nursing practice as well as generate different propositions that can later be used for research. For example, the assumption that the reduction of specific stressors, such as noise, within a hospital setting increases a person's line of resistance in relation to his emotional response can be validated if correct. Thus the theory serves a useful purpose for practice, and future research and could be predictive.

CALLISTA ROY:
DESCRIPTON OF THE THEORY

Roy's theory, which she views as a model at this stage of development, focuses on a holistic person as an adaptive system. As she describes it in *Theory Construction in Nursing,* a system involves input, output, and a feedback process (p. 50). Living systems involve internal and external stress, are negentropic, and are composed of matter and energy. Living systems have subsystems which are generally arranged in a hierarchy and have a tendency toward dynamic balance. Roy's approach to systems is similar in many ways to both Parsons's and Von Bertalanffy's, as well as to the approaches of other nurse theorists such as Rogers, Neuman, and Johnson. The focus of Roy's theory on adaptation differentiates her theory from others.

Table 6-9 demonstrates that the assumptions drawn by Roy basically stem from Harry Helson's approach to adaptation. Both view adaptation as a process that occurs within living systems in their interaction with their environment for the purpose of survival, growth, and reproduction. Chin views the input in relation to the concepts of tension and stress, which represent forms of stimuli, as identified by Helson, Von Bertalanffy, and Roy. Dynamics related to living systems within the environment represent change or growth in force and intensity. The stimuli represent the input, the change is the process experienced by a living system, and the output and feedback mechanisms relate to adaptation. Within the living system, the regulator and cognator subsystems provide ways of adapting. The regulator relates to physiological needs, and the cognator to self-concept, role cues, and interdependence.

Roy has developed propositions related to each subsystem. For example, under the *regulator* subsystem the following proposition is offered:

> Target organs or tissues must be able to respond to hormone levels to effect body response. (*Theory Construction in Nursing*)

The following proposition is related to the *cognator* subsystem:

Table 6-9

Assumptions within Roy's Adaptation Model, and Related Theories

Systems Theories	Helson's Adaptations Theory (1964)	Roy's Model (1976)
Chin (1961) The dynamics of a living system include observations about tension, stress, strain, and conflict. Systems have a feedback process. Parsons (1968) Individuals, as a unit within a system, have subsystems, which are the personality, the behavioral organism, and the social and cultural system. An open system has interchanging outputs and inputs. Von Bertalanffy (1968) Systems are sets "of elements standing in interaction." Every living thing is an open system. Feedback systems include a stimulus-receptor, a control apparatus, and an effector/response.	Adaptation is reflective of changes in the environment as influenced by stimulation. Adaptation is a product of both internally and externally initiated energies, and is a dynamic process. Problem, perception, affectivity, learning, cognition, and interpersonal relations conceived as modes of adaptation to focal, contextual, and residual stimuli.	The person's adaptation level is a function of focal, contextual, and residual stimuli. Changing environments demand a positive response in order for adaptation to occur. Both innate and acquired mechanisms are used to cope with a changing world. The modes of adaptation are physiological needs, self-concept, role function, and interdependence. Adaptive system includes stimuli, regulators, effectors, adaptive modes, and output, with a feedback system between input and output.

Intact pathways and perceptual/information processing apparatus positively influence the adequacy of selective attention, coding, and memory. (*Theory Construction in Nursing*)

These subsystems are thought to be connectives that link together the adaptive modes, physiological needs, self-concept, role function, and interdependence.

The various components within this theory in relation to the basic concepts are as follows:

Human/individual—an adaptive system with two mechanisms, the cognator and regulator, which function through adaptive modes—physiological, self-concept, role function, and interdependence.

Environment—Stimuli of the following three types arise from the internal and external environment: focal—the immediate degree of change/stimuli; contextual—other stimuli present; residual—attitudes and traits that affect the situation.

Health-Illness—one dimension of a person's total life experience, ranging from peak wellness to death.

Nursing—Practice-centered discipline oriented toward persons and how they respond to stimuli and adapt to the environment.

Roy's conceptual approach to health as shown in Figure 6-12, is based on a health-illness continuum, at one end of which is peak wellness, and at the other, death. Individuals move along this continuum based on their ability to handle stimuli from the environment and adapt to change.

From a holistic framework, it is difficult to place an individual at any exact point on the continuum. An individual who has a slight

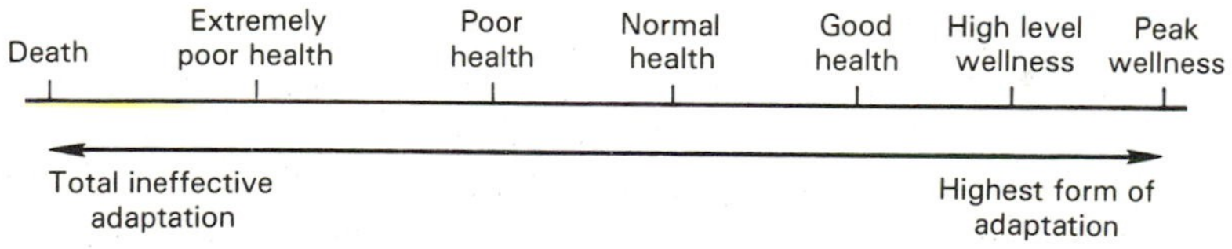

Figure 6-12. Roy's health-illness continuum. From Sister Callista Roy, "Adaptation as a Model of Nursing Practice", in *Introduction to Nursing: An Adaptation Model*, edited by Sister Callista Roy, © 1976, p. 18. Reprinted by permission of Prentice-Hall, Inc., Englewood Cliffs, N.J.

hearing problem and refuses a hearing aid might be considered to be in poor health since the lack of a hearing aid would influence the ability to deal with stimuli. On the other hand, an individual who has lost a leg but has adjusted very well to stimuli might be viewed as having a very high level of wellness. Attitudes, not physical condition, may have more influence on health status. The continuum implies that we can categorize all individuals based on seven levels, but this is purely an assumption that has not been validated.

Model

The concept of adaptation integrates these basic concepts into the model which Roy presents as shown in Figure 6-13.

Person as an Adaptive System

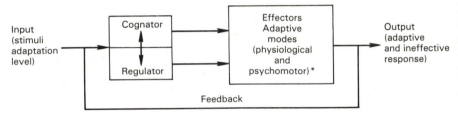

*-added for clarity (*Theory Construction in Nursing* p. 58)

Figure 6-13. From Sister Callista Roy, "Adaptation as a Model of Nursing Practice" in *Introduction to Nursing: An Adaptation Model,* edited by Sister Callista Roy, © 1976, p. 58. Reprinted by permission of Prentice-Hall, Inc., Englewood Cliffs, N.J.

The model is typical of systems models in its framework and can be used in relation to any of the four modes of adaptation.

The major concepts within Roy's theory can be broken down into the following three categories that relate to systems theory: (1) input—the focal, contextual, and residual stimuli, (2) process—the cognitive, regulative, and four adaptive modes, and (3) output—the adaptive and ineffective responses.

The *focal stimulus* is the predominant stimulus that is immediately confronting an individual; this may be viewed as the primary stressor. The *contextual stimuli* are the background or other factors present as related to the focal stimuli. The *residual stimuli* are related to the contextual stimuli because they also have an effect on the focal stimuli, but they are more difficult to assess or control; they include, for example, the beliefs, attitudes, or characteristic patterns of an individual. As concepts, these stimuli range from the more empirical and inferential, such as high temperature or pain, to the more abstract, such as self-concept. The accuracy of the assignment of a stimulus to these abstract categories is not very significant as long as the impact of all the presenting stimuli are taken into account.

Within the process there are basically six concepts. The *cognator* is a system that is affected by stimuli related to perception, learning, judgments, and feelings. The *regulator* is a system affected by neutral and chemical-electrical impulses/stimuli. These systems are related to reflexes and body responses to hormonal changes, as well as to perception and memory as influenced, for example, by drugs.

There are four additional concepts under *process,* which represent the adaptive modes. (See Table 6-10.) The physiological mode is less abstract than the other three, which are *self-concept, role function,* and *interdependence.* These represent methods that the individual uses to adapt. Because the latter three, which are all psychosocial, are abstract and overlap a great deal, it may be difficult to clearly categorize different stimuli under them at any given time. If, for example, an individual has difficulty relating to others and feels lonely, it would be difficult to separate his self-concept from his perceived role and need for independence. A separation would be arbitrary rather than conclusive.

The concepts under *output—adaptation* and *ineffective response* —are quite abstract and are key to the entire theory. Characteristics of *adaptation* include the following: (1) an activity accomplished as individuals interact with their environment, (2) the goal for survival, growth, and mastery, and (3) adjustment to conditions. Concepts that are very similar to *adaptation* and assist in explaining its meaning are *accommodate, arrange, fit, harmonize, suit,* and *conform.* These terms have cultural implications and are time oriented.

The use of the major concepts follows, with one example for each of the adaptative modes.

In order to properly use the theory, it would be necessary to integrate all of these examples at one time. For example, an individual who is dehydrated, has a high temperature, requests assistance in taking fluids, and is confused may have difficulty accepting his sick role and being dependent on the nurse. This example incorporates all four modes as well as the influence of the regulator and the cognator.

Within the theory, various specific concepts and propositions are provided by Roy and Roberts relating to each of the adaptive modes. This provides increased clarity as to the meaning of the major con-

Table 6-10

Roy's Adaptive Modes Integrated
with Systems Theory

Mode	Input	Process	Output
Temperature Physiological needs	High temperature; *Focal stimuli*—dehydration; *Contextual stimuli*—reduce physical activity; *Residual stimuli*—influence of previous experiences with high temperature	*Regulator*—subsystem attempts to maintain normal temperature → *Mode* *Physiological*—response of temperature-controlling mechanism, manipulate stimuli, provide fluids	*Adaptive* Maintain normal temperature; Ineffective response—continued high temperature
Self-concept Psychosocial mode	Feelings of inadequacy; *Focal stimuli*—lacks information about condition; *Contextual stimuli*—confusion; *Residual stimuli*—attitude toward authority figure	*Cognator*—ability to decide with inconsistency and lack of data → *Mode* *Self-concept*—provide clear information when available	*Adaptive* Accepts information and reduces state of confusion; Remain confused

Feedback

Feedback

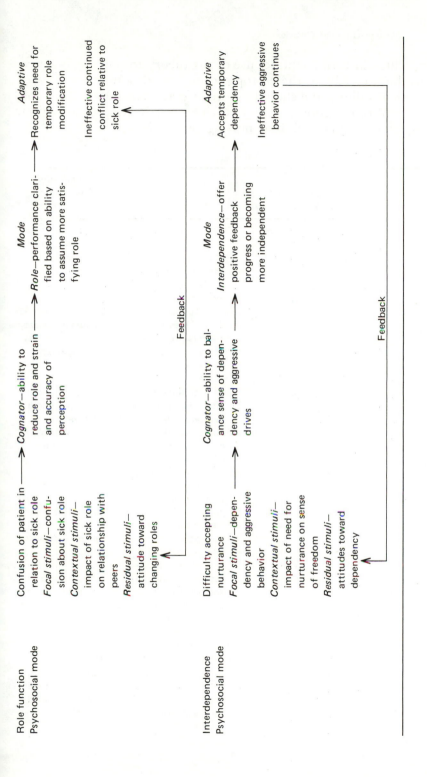

Role function Psychosocial mode

Confusion of patient in relation to sick role
Focal stimuli—confusion about sick role
Contextual stimuli—impact of sick role on relationship with peers
Residual stimuli—attitude toward changing roles

⟶ *Cognator*—ability to reduce role and strain and accuracy of perception

⟶ *Mode*
Role—performance clarified based on ability to assume more satisfying role

⟶ *Adaptive*
Recognizes need for temporary role modification

Ineffective continued conflict relative to sick role

Feedback

Interdependence Psychosocial mode

Difficulty accepting nurturance
Focal stimuli—dependency and aggressive behavior
Contextual stimuli—impact of need for nurturance on sense of freedom
Residual stimuli—attitudes toward dependency

⟶ *Cognator*—ability to balance sense of dependency and aggressive drives

⟶ *Mode*
Interdependence—offer positive feedback progress or becoming more independent

⟶ *Adaptive*
Accepts temporary dependency

Ineffective aggressive behavior continues

Feedback

cepts, which in turn facilitates use of the theory for nursing practice.
It must be realized that these propositions provide a base for research
to test their validity and should not be seen as empirical truths. Table
6-11 identifies the concepts under each mode, the propositions given
by Roy and Roberts, and some nursing implications.

Table 6-11

Adaptive Mode	Concepts (under each mode)	Propositions	Implication for Nursing Situations
Physiological needs	Exercise and rest	The amount of mobility in the form of exercising positively influences the level of muscle integrity.	The patient is encouraged to turn frequently in bed.
	Nutrition	An environment conducive to eating will positively influence the level of anorexia or nausea.	The patient is encouraged to eat in a community dining room.
	Elimination	The magnitude of internal and external stimuli will positively influence the level of urinary and intestinal elimination.	Increased fluid intake will stimulate urinary and intestinal elimination.
	Fluid and electrolytes	The level of hydration achieved will positively influence the level of fluid and electrolyte balance.	The patient drinks one glass of fluid at three-hour intervals to maintain fluid levels.
	Oxygen and circulation	The level of alveolar-capillary exchange and perfusion will positively influence the level of oxygenation and circulatory balance.	The patient is encouraged to do deep breathing exercises.
	Temperature	The amount of input in the form of heat will positively influence the temperature regulatory system.	The patient is provided with blankets at night to keep warm.

Table 6-11 (cont.)

Adaptive Mode	Concepts (under each mode)	Propositions	Implication for Nursing Situations
	The senses	The amount of sensory input via each sensory modality will positively influence the level of cortical arousal.	The noise and odors in the room are kept at an optimum level.
	Endocrine system	The amount of hormonal input and control will positively influence hormonal balance.	The nurse monitors the amount of sugar excreted in the patient's urine.
Psychosocial modes	Self-concept	Adequacy of role taking positively influences the level of feelings of adequacy.	The nurse assists a new father to understand his child's behavior.
	Role-function	The amount of clarity of input in the form of role cues positively influences the level of role mastery.	The nurse and the patient clearly identify the impact the patient's illness has on his vocational role.
	Interdependence	The optimum amount of environmental changes positively influence interdependence.	The patient is provided with mechanical devices that facilitate independence.

Application to Nursing Process

The use of the nursing process for Roy is similar to its use by other nurse theorists, except that there is a two-level approach to assessment that integrates the stimuli (input) with the adaptive modes and the two systems (process). Evaluation (output) is expressed in terms of the level to which the patient does or does not adapt (see Table 6-12). Basically, the major goal is to manipulate or influence the stimuli in such a way that the patient can achieve the highest possible level of adaptation within a changing environment. Thus, health, which is viewed on a continuum, is facilitated through adaptation.

The assessment phase requires an in-depth understanding of the patient's behaviors and responses to the environment, taking into account the influence of past experiences on the present. Also involved is how the patient is coping or adapting to the stimuli/stress that is constantly occurring within the environment. The specific stimuli that are most significant to the individual at any given time must be identified. This prioritization may lead to an emphasis on the focal stimuli that are classified under the physiological mode, neglecting the impact of psychological stimuli. It is possible that one could become involved in a comprehensive physiological study incorporating all the physiological needs and a complete personality study to understand the psychosocial needs. This is not realistic, however, and it is basically the emphasis on the focal stimuli that provides the nurse with the data to establish priorities.

The diagnosis needs to be made within a holistic framework. Thus, either a diagnosis that cuts across all the adaptive modes needs to be identified, or multiple diagnoses relating to several adaptive modes must be developed. Unless the diagnosis is thus developed, the care provided may be too limited to achieve the goal of adaptation. In the development of the plan, priorities again need to be identified, because the nurse cannot always deal in a given period of time with the number or the scope of the problems identified. Constant deduction is necessary in order to decide which specific implementation strategies will be most effective in enhancing adaptation. Further stimuli will be recognized during evaluation, so additional assessment data is collected and diagnoses are either further confirmed or eliminated based on the degree to which the patient has adapted. The ultimate goal of the use of the nursing process and Roy's theory is to achieve peak wellness in adapting to an ever-changing environment.

Evaluation

Roy's theory involves multiple concepts that are basically supportive of the ideas of Helson and the systems theorists. These concepts provide a framework with which to view the patient at some level of health/illness in relation to stimuli and the patient's ability to adapt. Most of the concepts are abstract and lack adequate definition and clarity. Thus the model can only be used in nursing practice with much interpretation, which may or may not be reflective of Roy's thinking.

Roy emphasizes a holistic approach to the patient and an open

Table 6-12

Nursing Process and Roy's Theory

	Structure of Nursing Process Assessment	Diagnosis	Plan	Implementation	Evaluation (output)
First Level	Cognator/Regulator systems > Effectiveness-adaptation > Physiological needs, Psychosocial modes	Statement of adaptive or ineffective response to stimuli.	Express goal setting in terms of resulting behavior expected on the part of the patient that facilitates adaptation.	Manipulate situation to influence the patient's ability to handle the stimuli and adapt.	Judge effectiveness of nursing intervention in relation to patient's ability to adapt.
Second Level	Stimuli: Behavior—focal —contextual —residual				

Limited implementation of nursing process in a clinical situation: Ms. Dunn enters the emergency room with her ten-year-old boy, Tim, who has been beaten by his father and complains of pain in his left shoulder. Tim is crying, withdrawn, and is hesitant to allow the physician to touch him.

	Structure of Nursing Process Assessment	Diagnosis	Plan	Implementation	Evaluation (output)
First Level	Gather information about the child's ability to move his left arm and shoulder, and to adjust to his father's violence, his mother's role as a support system, and his developmental level in terms of independence.	Difficulty moving left shoulder and caring for himself. Inability to effectively deal with father's violence. Pain due to trauma.	Provide opportunity for Tim to express himself and deal with feelings. Reduce pain and support shoulder.	Communicate with Ms. Dunn and Tim. Medication for pain. Brace shoulder.	Reassess Tim's ability to handle pain and deal with his feelings.
Second Level	Assess the degree of physical and emotional pain, the significance of his immobility on his activities, and his feelings about violence and about his father.				

system reflective of an environment that is constantly impacting the patient. The model implies, however, that individuals can be viewed from four adaptive modes that are *not* holistic and can reach some final state of adaptation. Open systems are dynamic and changing, not oriented toward stasis.

There is a lack of clarity as to the relationship between adaptation and the health–illness continuum. The degree of adaptation

Table 6-13

Characteristics of Systems Theory
and Specific Nursing Theories

Character-istic	Chin—1961	Parsons—1968	Von Berta-lanffy—1968	Johnson—1968
Basic concept	All living systems as open systems	Personality is an open system within the environment	General systems theory and open system	Systems evolve into subsystems which are linked and open
Organization	Organization, interdependency, and integration exist among the parts of the system.	Organization of personality into four subsystems of: personality, behavioral, social, and cultural. This is a pattern-maintaining approach.	Organization with wholeness, growth, differentiation, hierarchical order, dominance, control, competition.	Man's response patterns from an organized and integrated whole. Systems grow and develop.
Component elements	Tensions, stresses, or strains arise out of the structured arrangements of the system.	Subsystems have dynamic interactions.	Elements in mutual interaction.	Behavioral systems determine and limit the interaction between person and environment.
Direction/purpose/goal	Adjustment and adaptation is the goal.	Develop an identity system to gain meaning for the individual.	Adaptiveness, purposiveness, and goal seeking.	"Behavioral system reflects adjustments and adaptations that are successful in some way and to some degree."

as it relates to a person's state of health is unclear. Thus, the goal of nursing—to assist a person in adapting or coping—is difficult to implement.

The theory, if it had greater clarity, would not be too difficult to understand or utilize if one had an adequate scientific background and a knowledge of systems theory. Most of the words are familiar and have not been coined.

Rogers—1970	King—1971	Neuman—1972	Roy—1976
Man is open system	Human beings are open systems	Individual is open system	Person is open system
Pattern and organization identify man and reflect wholeness.	Major concepts are interaction, perception, communication, transaction, self, role, stress, growth, development, time, space.	Total-person model to maintain a degree of harmony and balance between external and internal environment.	A person is an adaptive system with adaptive mode of physiological needs, self-concept, role function, and interdependence.
Man and environment exchange matter and energy.	Humans interact with environment.	Individuals interact with environment and are composed of four variables: physiological, psychological, sociocultural, developmental.	Living systems exchange energy and matter with the environment and are affected by stimuli.
Life process includes probabilistic goal directedness.	Adjustments are influenced by individuals' interactions with environment. Nurse-client interactions lead to achievement of goals.	Within the environment, individuals adjust themselves to it or adjust the environment to themselves.	Adaptive responses promote the goal of survival, growth, reproduction, and self-mastery.

Although this theory focuses on the individual, with creativity it can be utilized to deal with families and with the community. Roy's theory can also be used in multiple settings, not just in acute care settings.

SUMMARY OF SYSTEMS THEORY

Systems theories have gained increasing attention across disciplines during the last twenty years. Nursing theorists and researchers in greater numbers are moving toward a systems approach and away from a need orientation. A systems framework is more complex, because it tends to involve concepts that are more abstract and difficult to understand.

There are basic similarities among almost all the systems theories presented, from Chin's to Roy's. In reviewing systems theories (Table 6-13), the following should be evident:

1. Human beings are an open system; thus, the individual constantly interacts with the environment, and there are many variables that must be accounted for at any given time.
2. The feedback system incorporates the dynamic nature of the system.
3. Systems have organization, patterns, and integration, and are reflective of wholeness.
4. The direction in the utilization of systems theory involves adjustment/adaptation or nonspecific goal achievement.

The interpretation or specific process for utilization of these generalizations differs among the theorists. Chin's orientation moves toward using systems theory to deal with change within an institution. Johnson uses systems through a behavioral approach, and King focuses on the interaction, emphasizing perception. Chin, Parsons, Roy, and Neuman view the organization of a system as having parts. Rogers would view this as a contradiction to an open-system approach and focuses on total pattern and wholeness. Some theorists, such as King, provide more specific characteristics of the individual and explanations of the meaning of the concepts, while others, such as Rogers, offer fewer.

The concepts related to (1) *inputs* are *stress, energy,* and *matter, perception,* and *stimuli,* (2) *process* are *dynamic stability, energy field, resources, interpersonal systems,* or *modes,* and (3) *output* are *adaptation, changing the form of energy and information, goal achievement,* and *reconstitution.* These concepts have similarities as well as differences, which give the theories a somewhat different focus. More detailed definitions/characteristics of these concepts would be needed in order to enable a clearer understanding of their meanings so that research could be carried out to identify the significance of their differences.

The major concepts reflected within all systems theories are *human/individual* and his *relationship with the environment.* Limited emphasis is placed on the concept of *nurse*; that emphasis was more common among the need theorists. Also, the concept of *health* is not well developed, except by inference, among the nursing need and systems theorists. As a matter of fact, among the four major concepts in nursing, *health* remains the most abstract and poorly understood.

REFERENCES

Bennes, W.G., K.D. Benne and R. Chin. *The Planning of Change,* 2d ed. New York: Holt, Rinehart & Winston, 1969.

Chin, R. "The Utility of Systems, Models and Developmental Models For Practitioners." In *Conceptual Models for Nursing Practitioners,* 2d ed., edited by J.P. Riehl and C. Roy. New York: Appleton-Century-Crofts, 1980.

Helson, H. *Adaptation Level Theory.* New York: Harper and Row Publishers, Inc., 1964.

Johnson, D.E. "The Behavioral System For Nursing," In *Conceptual Models for Nursing Practice,* 2d ed., edited by J.P. Riehl and C. Roy, pp. 207–216. New York: Appleton-Century-Crofts, 1980.

King, I.M. *A Theory of Nursing: Systems, Concepts, Process.* New York: John Wiley & Sons, Inc., 1981.

Neuman, B. *The Neuman Systems Model: Application to Nursing Education and Practice.* East Norwalk, Conn.: Appleton-Century-Crofts, 1982.

Parsons, T. "The Position of Identity in General Theory of Action." In *Self in Social Interaction,* by G. Chase and G. Kennult, pp. 11–13. John Wilson & Son Co. Chattanooga, Tenn., 1968.

Rogers, M.E. *An Introduction to the Theoretical Basis of Nursing.* Philadelphia: F.A. Davis Company, 1970.

Roy, C., and S. Roberts. *Theory Construction in Nursing; An Adaptation Model.* Englewood Cliffs, N.J.: Prentice-Hall, Inc., 1981.

von Bertalanffy, L. *General System Theory.* New York: George Braziller, Inc., 1968.

7

THEORIES ORIENTED TOWARD
THE INTERACTION PROCESS

INTRODUCTION

The major emphasis of interaction-oriented nursing theories is the *relationship* between the patient and the nurse and the results of that relationship, especially its effect on the patient. The characteristics of the patient and the nurse are thought to have an impact on the interaction, affecting the outcome. The theories that are foundational to the interactive approaches are basically psychological in nature, like those of Harry Sullivan and Carl Rogers. Learning theories, such as John Dewey's, also provide a base for the interpersonal approaches aimed toward educating patients about their behavior. Dewey stressed the importance of judging the learning process in terms of outcome, especially the continued desire to learn.

Whether one focuses on nursing, teaching, social work, or other service professions, the emphasis is on interaction. For purposes of this chapter, Carl Rogers's work will be reviewed as the basis for the interactive nursing theories, recognizing that many other non-nurse theorists have affected the nurse theorists. It should also be understood that other nursing theorists, such as Orlando (a need theorist) and King (a systems theorist), describe nursing as interactive, and as requiring effective communication. Actually all nurse theorists, some more than others, relate to the interaction of the nurse with the patient and its effect on the goal of care.

HISTORICAL DEVELOPMENT

A Frame of Reference—Nurse ⟵interaction⟶ Patient

During the early 1950s, psychiatrists and psychologists were taking a closer look at the interaction between the client and the therapist. This prompted nursing theorists to focus on the patient-nurse relationship as a therapeutic force. The historical development as shown in Table 7-1 reflects a consistent interest in further explaining the meaning of the interaction.

Table 7-1

Historical Development of Interaction Theories

Theory		Major Theme
Carl Rogers	1942 and 1951	Client-centered therapy is a process involving achievement by the individual in terms of growth and maturational development from the time of conception onward.
Peplau	1951–52	Nursing is a therapeutic, interpersonal process which, as an educational instrument, aims to promote the forward movement of the personality for productive living within the community.
Hall	1962	Nursing uses interpersonal skills and reflective techniques, acting like a mirror for the patient to explore feelings.
Levine	1966	Nursing is a human interaction involving communication rooted in the organic dependency of the individual on his relationship with others.
Travelbee	1971	Nursing is an interpersonal process in which the nurse assists individuals, families, and the community to prevent or cope with the experience of illness and suffering and find meaning in these experiences.
Watson	1979	Nursing (which is practiced interpersonally) is based on a scientific-humanistic base which is used in a caring process.

CARL ROGERS

In his *Counseling and Psychotherapy* (1942) and *Client-Centered Therapy* (1951), Rogers focuses on the need for the counselor to understand her own attitudes, the therapeutic relationship as experienced by the client, and the process of therapy. The basic approach is nondirective, incorporating the counselor's understanding and acceptance of the client's private world. The relationship must include emotional warmth, respect, empathy, acceptance, and safety. The client's perception of himself and his world is utilized by the counselor as the focus of the interaction. The therapist as a separate person keeps her own interpretation of reality, which may be distorted, out of the interactive process if at all possible, which results in a greater understanding of the client. This frees clients to explore their lives and experiences in depth, finding new meanings and new goals.

Rogers provides certain propositions that he perceives as theory building. They focus on the individual's characteristics and behaviors. These propositions focus on some major concepts of the theory, such as *change, perception, organized whole, self-enhancement needs, conflict/tension, interaction,* and *symbolism.* The following statements can be drawn from these propositions and characterize Rogers's view of individuals:

1. The individual's perceived world is his reality.
2. Individuals have the tendency to actualize, maintain, and enhance themselves in a changing environment.
3. An individual reacts as an organized whole in order to satisfy his perceived needs.
4. Individuals experience life through symbolism as it relates to their self-concepts.
5. Individuals interact with the environment with differing intensity of emotion depending upon the significance of the event to their self-maintenance and enhancement.
6. Tension/conflict is created when there is a discrepancy between an individual's world and the symbolic world of others who are perceived as well adjusted.

Rogers identifes the characteristics of an ideal client-counselor relationship. The most important one is the therapist's ability to participate completely in the patient's communication. Other characteristics include the following:

—The counselor's comments closely relate to what the client is trying to convey. The counselor reinforces the client's perception of reality in such a way that the client acknowledges the accuracy of the comments.

—The counselor sees the client as a co-worker on a common

problem. This statement supports the idea that the client is truly involved in the therapeutic process and is not merely the receiver of the counselor's input.

—The counselor treats the client as an equal. This facilitates respect on the part of the counselor for the client and enhances communication.

—The counselor tries and is able to understand the client's feelings. The entire focus is on the client's feelings, which the counselor accepts as his perception.

—The line of thought during the counseling sessions is the client's. Again the emphasis is completely client centered.

—The counselor's tone of voice conveys the complete ability to share the client's feelings. This facilitates a nonjudgmental attitude on the part of the counselor about what the client is saying and feeling.

The client is to experience the therapeutic relationship as a process. This process is viewed by Rogers as an experience of responsibility, of *exploration,* of the *discovery* of *denied attitudes,* of *reorganizing* the self, and of *progress* and *ending.* This could be viewed as a six-step process oriented toward both the client's and counselor's accepting termination of the relationship when the problem has been adequately dealt with by the client. As you will note later in the chapter, Peplau uses similar steps in her theory.

With the goal of behavioral changes in the direction of improved adjustment, Rogers offers the following, based on research, as a way of evaluating the success of the client-centered approach:

—There is a decrease in psychological tension as evidenced in the communication.

—The client shows increased tolerance for frustration as indicated in physiological terms.

—The client's behaviors move from relatively immature to relatively mature in nature.

—The client appears less defensive in his behaviors and has a greater awareness of such behaviors.

—The client increasingly discusses plans and behavioral steps to be undertaken in relation to identified outcomes.

—There is improved functioning in life tasks, such as job performance.

Rogers philosophically believes that humans/clients are trustworthy organisms, capable of evaluating their inner and outer situations, making constructive choices, and acting on those choices. Counselors relate as real persons, owning and expressing their own feelings, being nonpossessive in their caring, and accepting the inner world of others. This kind of relationship leads to choice and actions that are increasingly constructive to both the client and the counselor and tend to create a more realistic social harmony. Thus, the client and the counselor have much to gain by this nondirective, client-centered interpersonal process.

HILDEGARD PEPLAU: DESCRIPTION OF THE THEORY

The major concepts of Peplau's theory are the *individual,* the *nurse,* and the *interactive* process. *Nursing* is defined as a human relationship between an individual who is sick or in need of health service and the nurse. The goal of this relationship is the achievement of health through the use of an interpersonal nursing process as a maturing and educating force which leads patients to develop skills in problem solving. *Health* is viewed as a symbol that implies the force and movement of the personality toward creative, constructive, and productive personal and community living. Interacting conditions essential for health are both physiological and interpersonal. Peplau focuses on the interpersonal process and its relationship to facilitating interpersonal health. Thus, of the four main concepts of nursing, Peplau relates most strongly to *human* and *nursing. Health* is only superficially dealt with, and *environment* is viewed in a limited way from the perspective of its impact on the relationship (see Figure 7-1).

Nurses are assumed to have many roles; the nurse is a consultant, tutor, safety agent, mediator, administrator, recorder, and observer. The nurse enters the interpersonal relationship as a stranger, with respect and a positive interest in the patient. The nurse is a resource person who provides information, teaches the patient, and acts as a leader in a democratic manner.

Humans have personalities oriented toward growth and development and needs. Immediate needs, when met, lead to more mature needs. Needs create tension, and behaviors are oriented toward reducing this tension. Peplau supports Maslow's premise that it is essential to meet basic needs before higher needs can be met.

The nurse-patient interpersonal relationship is characterized by four overlapping phases—*orientation, identification, exploitation,* and *resolution.* Each phase has tasks and roles that are required of both the nurse and the patient and that enter into every nursing situation (see Table 7-2).

The four stages, which are very similar to Rogers's six experiences, are related to the nursing process. As in the nursing process, the steps are not clearly defined or rigidly sequential. Orientation

Table 7-2

Peplau's Interpersonal Phases

Nurse Role ————————➤	Interpersonal Phases (Nursing Process) ◄————————	Patient Role
Professional help to be provided. Identify role. Gather observable objective data. Identify peripheral or subproblems. Encourage patient to be an *active* partner through orientation. Assist patient in recognizing and planning to use professional services. Know own pattern in establishing relationship.	*Orientation* (assessment, diagnoses, and plan) Mutually recognize, clarify, define existing problem/felt need.	Experience a "felt need." Recognize difficulty and extent of need for help. Plan to use professional services. Use energy created from harnessed tension to define and understand problem. Clarify impression of the problem. Participate in orientation process by observing and questioning.
Permit patient to express what he feels to reorient feelings and strengthen positive forces in personality. Allow expression of helplessness, self-centeredness, dependency. Assist during stress. Symbolize acceptance.	*Identification* (assessment, diagnoses, and plan) Patient responds selectively to people who can meet his needs.	Respond to persons who offer help in relation to identified needs. Explore feelings. Participate in an interdependent relationship with the nurse rather than isolation or dependence on the nurse.
Assist patient in their efforts to strike a balance between a a need to be dependent and a need to be independent. Understand that awareness of feelings can cause severe anxiety.	*Exploitation* (implementation) Patient uses all services available.	Derive full value from the relationship by realistically exploiting resources based on self-interest and need.
Assist patient to be free for more productive social activities and relationships.	*Resolution* (evaluation) Patient needs are met.	Put old needs aside willingly. Formulate new goals. Relinquish dependencies.

and identification are being practiced almost constantly, but they are most used during the assessment, diagnosis, and planning stages. Exploitation relates most to implementation, and resolution most to evaluation. In using these phases, Peplau identifies two types of counseling—immediate situational counseling and developmental counseling. During an immediate counseling situation the nurse helps the patient to describe, analyze, and formulate an immediate response to the current situation. Developmental counseling evolves when a long-term nurse-patient relationship is needed for the promotion of self-understanding and learning about living through the use of illness as an experience that has meaning.

Peplau is oriented toward meeting human needs, recognizing that needs are physiological as well as psychological. She views the need for rest, food, and drink as being as important as the need for prestige and power. Humans as organisms have an unstable equilibrium and a drive toward stability.

Peplau supports Rogers's nondirective techniques which permit the direction and content to be determined by the patient within a permissive environment. Rapport established through trust, respect, and shared satisfaction in an empathic atmosphere is viewed as an essential component of the relationship.

Model

This model, which represents Peplau's major concepts, is basically linear and directional. The central focus is on the interpersonal phases of the nurse-patient relationship. The environment has an im-

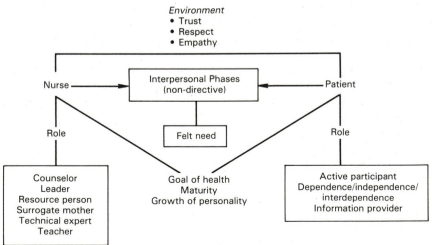

Figure 7-1. Peplau model.

pact on the nurse and patient, who have an impact on the goal of health. The roles of the nurse and the patient impact on each of them and on the interpersonal process.

Application to the Nursing Process

The situation described in Table 7-3, although it reflects a very brief encounter with a patient's visitor, provides a framework with which to view nursing situations. Based on the model, the nurse's role is that of counselor and the visitor's is that of active participant seeking independence. The interpersonal relations reflected mutual respect. The nurse was empathetic as she encouraged the visitor to sit down and immediately discuss her need. The goal of the interaction was to help the visitor to identify for herself a way of helping herself, which is a maturing force. The nurse also recognized her ability to assist a patient through an effective interaction with the visitor. Later, the nurse can use this information to communicate with the patient about his needs.

Evaluation

This descriptive theory is basically process oriented rather than strongly theoretical. The four major concepts are included, with *health* as the goal of nursing care. Certain assumptions are basic to the theory, although they are not always clearly stated. For example, *humans* are viewed as having the capacity to play multiple roles and to be empathic in a trusting relationship. A positive *environment* facilitates communication and problem solving. *Health* is represented by the level of maturity achieved as patients experience stress in relation to their needs. These assumptions help clarify the meaning of the concepts but do not adequately define their meaning.

The process utilized within the theory, which describes the nurse-patient interaction in different phases, does provide a different frame of reference with which to practice nursing. Neither the disease, nor the nurse, nor the physician is the central focus of the theory. The relationship, activity, and communication, verbal and nonverbal, are the essence of the theory. This process as described by Peplau is abstract and unclear, which is probably true about the definitions of most psychological terms or communication activities. As you will note in the remainder of this chapter, interpersonal/interaction theories are quite abstract and require much individual interpretation, as was evident in Carl Rogers's theory.

Table 7-3

Limited Situation—A visitor enters the nursing unit expressing a need for help in relation to the sudden illness of her brother.

Patient Visitor	Nurse	Major Interpersonal Process and Comments
Could someone help me?	Hello, I'm Miss Stanton. How can I help you?	*Orientation*—Patient's visitor acknowledges need for help; nurse is viewed as a counseling person.
My brother has just had a heart attack, and I'm not sure I can cope.	Let's sit down together and talk about it.	Nurse makes observations and communicates with the visitor.
Do you have time?	Yes I do.	Nurse plans to provide immediate counseling and reassures visitor that she wants to help her.
I feel so anxious. My brother and I have lived together for many years, and he takes care of all the money and the house. It seems that lately everything is going wrong.	Tell me what is happening.	Nurse seeks further clarification of the problem.
My brother lost his job last week, and I haven't worked in several years. I'm not sure how we'll make ends meet. I feel so helpless.	You feel helpless in relation to your inability to survive economically. What do you think you need to do?	*Identification*—Nurse permits visitor to be helpless and self-centered, tries to understand the visitor's concerns, and facilitates her ability to help herself.
Yes, I need to survive economically. I have worked as a secretary and was good at it. Guess I'll need to go to the employment agency I used before.	That sounds like a good idea.	*Exploitation*—Nurse recognizes visitor's need to become independent and provides positive feedback.
Thanks a lot of listening. My brother will be happy to hear of my plans.	Let me know if there is anything else you need.	*Resolution*—Visitor's immediate needs have been met.
I'll see you tomorrow if you have time and let you know how I did.	Fine.	Visitor no longer views the nurse as a stranger.

The terms used in the phases of the interpersonal process are descriptive in nature and do not seem to be coined by Peplau. *Orientation* means the process of being intellectually or emotionally directed. *Identification*, in psychological terms, relates to feeling a close emotional association with others for gratification, emotional support, or relief from stress. *Exploitation* means taking advantage of a resource for one's gain or advantage. *Resolution* involves finding an answer to or reaching a firm decision about something. These basic definitions support Peplau's explanations about the use of the terms.

Although Peplau acknowledges the existence of phases, the process is not linear, and many areas overlap. It is not clear what the relationship between the phases are. Questions such as the following arise: At what point in the relationship does orientation become less significant and identification take place? Does the resolution of a specific felt need lead to the termination of the relationship if the nurse identifies a further need and the patient does not recognize it? Is it possible that all four phases are occurring constantly and that no real separation exists in dealing with complex behaviors? Thus, the relationship between the phases as concepts is unclear. Admittedly, this may be unimportant in terms of practice if a therapeutic environment is created and the felt need is met.

The theory is not complex, especially if one has an adequate background in psychology and counseling theories. It incorporates such theories into the nursing situation.

LYDIA HALL:
DESCRIPTION OF THE THEORY

There are three major concepts to Hall's theory: the *care,* the *cure,* and the *core. Care* exclusively reflects the nurturance component of nursing. It involves intimate bodily care and is centered around biology and physiology. *Cure* is viewed as the medical aspect of nursing, oriented toward pathology/illness and treatment of disease. *Core* utilizes interpersonal/psychological approaches to nursing care. When these three concepts mesh or are integrated, total care can occur in the context of health promotion and maintenance. The differentiation between care, core, and cure demonstrates Hall's commitment to the differentiation between nursing and medicine. (See the model in Figure 7-2).

The theory relates to the four major concepts as follows. *Nursing* is an interpersonal nurturing and comforting process involving the laying on of hands. Nurses also assist physicians in some of their functions, but this is not their major role. When nurses deal with the medical/cure aspect of care, they participate in discomforting activi-

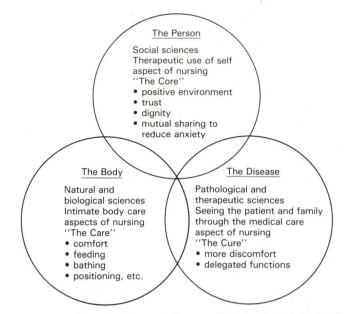

The Person

Social sciences
Therapeutic use of self
aspect of nursing
"The Core"
• positive environment
• trust
• dignity
• mutual sharing to
  reduce anxiety

The Body

Natural and
biological sciences
Intimate body care
aspects of nursing
"The Care"
• comfort
• feeding
• bathing
• positioning, etc.

The Disease

Pathological and
therapeutic sciences
Seeing the patient and family
through the medical care
aspect of nursing
"The Cure"
• more discomfort
• delegated functions

Figure 7-2. From Gertrude Torres, "Florence Nightingale," Julia B. George, "Lydia E. Hall," in *Nursing Theories: The Base for Professional Nursing Practice*, 2nd Ed., edited by Julia B. George, © 1985, pp. 41, 115. Reprinted by permission of Prentice-Hall, Inc., Englewood Cliffs, N.J.

ties, such as performing painful techniques. Nurses utilize themselves as therapeutic agents to facilitate the exploration of feelings when there is anxiety. *Humans,* who must be viewed as wholes, are the focus of nursing care. They have the capacity to learn to love others as themselves, become more self-accepting, and understand their feelings of anxiety. The *environment* is particularly important: It should be one that is accepting and nonjudgmental and in which there is trust. Thus, the emphasis is on the emotional interactive environment. *Health* is viewed as a goal when illness occurs. The emphasis is really on a nonhealth state—illness—which requires growth and rehabilitation on the part of the patient.

Model

Hall's model (Fig. 7-2) identifies three interacting circles which comprise the three main concepts of the theory. Essentially this is a model reflective of core identification. Each circle denotes an aspect of the nursing process related to the patient, the supporting science, and the underlying philosophical dynamics. The circles shown in Figure 7-2, which reflect an equal emphasis on the person, the body, and the disease, change in size depending upon the patient's progress and upon whether the physician, nurse, or patient has the major role in the rehabilitation. Table 7-4 shows some possible modifications of the three interacting circles and gives a statement showing the emphasis of each.

Table 7-4

Modified Model	Major Emphasis
1. Cure / Care / Core	The emphasis is on the medical care aspect of patient care—that of a disease orientation, with the nurse providing supportive care as developed by the physician. This modification is particularly true on, for example, the day of surgery. Note the limited involvement of the core aspect, because the patient is not alert or able to deal with his feelings. The model basically reflects the approach used in an acute care environment.
2. Core / Care / Cure	Here the interpersonal aspect is emphasized, with the patient and the nurse focusing on the psychological aspects of nursing care (Core). This model would be particularly important during a health-teaching experience. There is normal interaction with the physician and emphasis on medical orders. This model is more reflective of an environment that focuses on rehabilitation.
3. Care / Core / Cure	At times the major role of the nurse is nurturance, when intimate bodily care is essential. This might be true in the case of an elderly patient in a nursing home who is unable to communicate or perform his own personal care.

Each model must be reflective of the particular patient, the environment, and the goals of nursing care. This frame of reference helps to clarify the focus or central component of nursing care at any time. Each interaction with the patient may modify the particular emphasis. Thus, the nursing process is dynamic and constantly being modified to some degree.

The most significant impact Hall's theory has on the nursing process is the focus on the patient rather than on the nurse or on the physician. The theory supports the following *propositions/assumptions* in the practice of nursing.

1. The focus of nursing and medical care, which are distinct from each other, is on the patient, who experiences an illness.
2. Verbal and personal interactions enhance learning and growth (core).
3. Nursing care is both comforting (care) and discomforting (cure).
4. The biological (care) and psychological (core) condition of the patient has an impact on illness (cure).
5. Illness increases one's potential for self-awareness.
6. Both the patient and the nurse have the capacity to trust and share feelings (core).

The quality of nursing care is believed to range from not so good to very good. This could be viewed from the level of involvement of the patient as follows:

Low————————————Levels of patient involvement————————————High

Not so good ————————————————————————— Very good

against the patient / *at* the patient / *to* the patient / *for* the patient / *with* the patient

Since the emphasis is on the interpersonal process, quality nursing care is reflective of the nurse's functioning *with* the patient. Working *at* the patient can create a feeling of helplessness on the part of the patient and reflects a nursing approach that is oriented toward facilitating the nurse rather than the patient. Providing care *to* the patient creates a state of dependency and probably of physical comfort, and the patient feels like he has been in custody. An orientation toward providing care *for* patients increases patients' participation in their care because the nurse provides information relative to the care. The decisions within this approach are still the nurse's, because she perceives that she knows best. There is some increased independence on the part of patients, and they perceive that their feelings have been considered. Functioning *with* the patient is received as truly professional, rather than vocational, which is more the case with functioning *at* and *to* the patient. Here the emphasis is on the concept *core* and the *interpersonal process.* This can be modeled within the interpersonal process oriented toward Carl Rogers's theory.

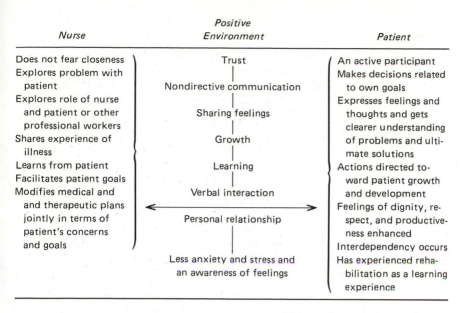

Nurse	Positive Environment	Patient
Does not fear closeness	Trust	An active participant
Explores problem with patient		Makes decisions related to own goals
	Nondirective communication	
Explores role of nurse and patient or other professional workers		Expresses feelings and thoughts and gets clearer understanding
	Sharing feelings	
Shares experience of illness	Growth	of problems and ultimate solutions
Learns from patient	Learning	Actions directed toward patient growth
Facilitates patient goals		and development
Modifies medical and and therapeutic plans jointly in terms of patient's concerns and goals	Verbal interaction	Feelings of dignity, respect, and productiveness enhanced
	Personal relationship	
		Interdependency occurs
	Less anxiety and stress and an awareness of feelings	Has experienced rehabilitation as a learning experience

Application to Nursing Process

Hall views nursing as an interpersonal process; she does not state specifically that it is a nursing process. She does not have Peplau's phases of relationship with which to compare the nursing process. The three main concepts and their relationship must be included within the nursing process as shown in Table 7-5.

Implied within any patient-centered nursing situation is the commitment of the nurse, physician, and other health care professionals to function as a team, facilitating one another's roles and functions so that the patient's goals can be met. In other words, all professionals focus on the patient through effective communication with one another. This practical approach was initiated at Loeb Center for Nursing and Rehabilitation in 1962. The center cared for patients who were in the stage of illness between the successful passing of a crisis and the returning to an optimum level of self-care. The center focused on such needs of patients as the needs to possess things of their own, to rest, to balance tension and relaxation, to receive praise, and to be listened to; this emphasis was described in an address by Lucile Petry Leone at the center's dedication ceremony in 1962. The environment in which this kind of nursing is practiced must also be patient oriented. The care provided centers around the

Table 7-5

Nursing Process	Patient-Centered Focus	Integration of Main Concepts
Assessment	Collect data for the benefit of the patient through interpersonal process (core). Identify needs/problems related to personal biological care (care). Facilitate collection of data related to physical condition, such as laboratory tests (care).	Measure patient's motivation to bathe self and accept medications.
Diagnosis	Statement of need/problem includes level of anxiety.	Anxiety due to impending surgery, and need to be dependent.
Plan	Establish patient-centered goals especially as related to rehabilitation and self-awareness.	Facilitate patient goal of independence in terms of feeding self. Identify impact of patient illness on family.
Implementation	Provide nurturance (care) with focus on interpersonal communication (core). Support medical regime (cure).	Use nondirective communication while bathing the patient and giving injections. Nurse and patient share understanding in terms of the need for cure.
Evaluation	Observation of the nursing process. Gather data related to the characteristics of nursing care. Review status of need, problem, and goal, especially in relationship to patient's learning to understand own feelings.	Observe nurse-patient interactions in terms of the level of anxiety. Review goals and motivations with the patient.

immediate recovery period after an acute illness. It would be difficult to practice Hall's theory in the environment of a hospital that was oriented toward diseases and the function of nurses rather than toward patient needs and goals.

Evaluation

The three major concepts differ from one another in level of abstraction. *Core* is the most abstract and is concerned with the interactive process, which is difficult to characterize specifically. Related terms are *trust, love, dignity,* and *anxiety,* which are also abstract. Aside from the notion of nondirective communication as viewed by Carl Rogers, there is little clarity as to how communication occurs. No directives or specific guidelines are offered, except for the identification of the nurse's role and the need for a positive environment in which interaction should occur.

Within the concept of *cure* are inferential indicators that can be utilized. Laboratory reports and physical assessment techniques, such as blood pressure monitoring, can be used to measure the extent of an illness and its impact on the patient. Since this concept is based on pathological conditions, the characteristics as developed by medical science have been identified. Thus the nurse, in performing functions directed by the physician, has a clearer sense of her role.

The *care* concept is also relatively inferential and easy to comprehend. It uses the characteristics of what is thought to be the nurturing/mothering aspect of nursing. Bathing, feeding, and moving are only a few of the activities/characteristics of this concept. Thus, *cure* and *care* are mostly empirical and inferential, while *core* is the most abstract and difficult to understand.

The assumptions/propositions that were developed from the theory are not complex or difficult to understand. They are logical and supportive of counseling and psychological theories, especially Carl Rogers's. The relationships between the major concepts within the model are clearly outlined so that propositions flow easily.

Although the theory identifies the patient as the focus in terms of needs and problems, there is no real explanation of what these specifically measure. The integration of need theories and interaction theories might be helpful.

This descriptive theory provides a frame of reference with which to practice nursing. Its major contribution in the early 1960s was its ability to separate nursing care as an art involving technique, medical care and its disease and treatment orientation, and the interpersonal process that facilitates problem solving.

MYRA ESTRIN LEVINE: DESCRIPTION OF THE THEORY

The major concepts incorporated into Levine's patient-centered care theory are *interaction/communication, internal* and *external patient environment, adaptation* and the *nurses' conservation principles. Humans* are viewed in a holistic manner from the perspective of their interaction with the environment. *Nursing* intervention focuses on the patient/nurse interaction, utilizing the four conservation principles. Nursing is therapeutic when adaptation is favorable and supportive when the status quo or reduced adaptation occurs. The *environment* is seen as internal and external. The internal environment is described using Walter Common's (1915) coined word *homeostates,* which describes the body's way of maintaining equilibrium in the face of constant change. This is Levine's approach to describing and understanding *health* and illness. *Adaptation* is the method of handling change in order to retain the integrity of the individual. Poor adaptation may create a different level of effectiveness and quality of life. The external environment is described by Bates in three categories as follows:

Perceptual—sense organs response to stimuli; for example, sight, sound, and order.

Operational—requires equipment to measure; examples include radioactivity, microorganisms, and air and water pollution.

Conceptual—relates to ideas, beliefs, tradition, and values.

The *interaction* is described as both verbal and nonverbal. The nurse must project a sense of certainty and knowledgeability as well as be attentive and prompt in meeting needs. Communication ranges from a casual social exchange to a complex teacher-learner relationship.

Model

The model shown in Figure 7-3 represents the relationship between the major concepts that emerges from Levine's definitions. Although she does not specifically provide a model, she writes in such a way that it is relatively easy to understand her ideas about the relationship of the major concepts and to develop a model. The following assumptions/propositions emerge deductively from her definitions and the developed model:

1. The patient and the nurse interact through verbal and nonverbal communication.
2. The patient is affected by the interaction of the internal and external environment.
3. The interaction between the internal and external environment affects the patient's ability to adapt.
4. The nurse utilizes the principles of conservation in the

interaction between the patient's internal and external environment.

The focus of this theory is the interactive process, both between the nurse and patient and between the internal and external environment of the patient.

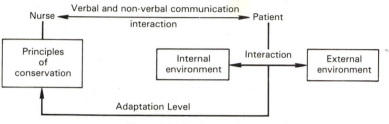

Figure 7-3. Levine model.

According to Levine, a principle provides a way of thinking and a structure for understanding nursing activities. These principles provide the formulation for the interaction that occurs between the nurse and the patient, and the goal is adaptation. The conservation principles are used by the nurse in relation to the ability of the patient to participate. There is a focus on helping the patient adapt by maintaining a proper balance between the activities of the patient and the nurse. The four principles relate to energy and to structural, personal, and social integrity. The latter three are reflective of the biological (structural), psychological (personal), and social framework in which most theorists view individuals (see Table 7-6).

Table 7-6

Framework for Conservation Principle

Wholeness of Individual			
Energy	Structural integrity	Personal integrity	Social integrity
Work	Anatomical and physiological structure	Sense of identity, self-worth, self-esteem	Social communities and relationships—family, friends
	Healing	Uniqueness as related to culture/religion	Isolation during hospitalization
		Sense of dependence	Social restrictions of hospital
		Self-image	Societal impacts
		Moral censure	Health care system

The principles basically include abstract concepts such as *energy,* and *personal and social integrity. Structural integrity* contains concepts that are mostly inferential, such as healing.

CONSERVATION OF ENERGY

Energy is not created or lost, but transforms from one kind to another. Energy is the ability to do work. Life processes involve the production and use of energy. There is an energy balance which the nurse must consider and which affects all nursing intervention. Disease processes create the need for greater energy, and rest is aimed at energy conservation.

CONSERVATION OF STRUCTURAL INTEGRITY

The structural integrity of human beings relates to anatomical and physiological wholeness and the healing process. The focus of nursing is to limit the amount of tissue involvement in infection and disease by identifying those activities that facilitate the healing process and minimize scarring.

CONSERVATION OF PERSONAL INTEGRITY

The individual is unique in his personal view of the world. Each person has a sense of identity and self-worth and is capable of decision making. The nurse must respect the patient, not make moral judgments, and must provide the patient with privacy.

CONSERVATION OF SOCIAL INTEGRITY

An individual needs to be viewed from the framework of his social life as reflected by family, friends, job, church, and the community as a social system. Illness is seen as a lonely, isolating event that creates new problems which must be resolved by the participation of the family and significant others.

These four principles of conservation aim at identifying the specific areas with which nurses must deal during interaction. In essence they describe the individual's characteristics from the framework of illness within the hospital environment. In dealing with an ill patient, the focus would be on such areas as ability to use energy, healing capacity, self-image, and relationship with the family. Levine believes that the medical diagnosis directs nursing care, which is basically related to the conservation area of structural integrity. She does not deal with emotional and psychiatric categories of disease, and the conservation areas of personal and social integrity are actually related to a health state requiring adaptation to illness. The model shown in Figure 7-4 is representative of a patient who is ill and is hospitalized. This experience can create a loss of structural integrity, leading to a greater need for energy, a loss of independence, and social isolation. The assumption is that when the structural integrity returns, energy is restored, there is less isolation, and adaption occurs. This sequence also implies that the nursing intervention has been therapeutic.

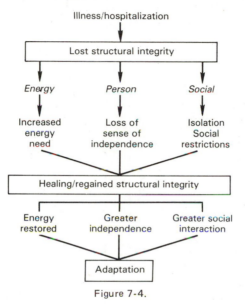

Figure 7-4.

Application to the Nursing Process

Levine believed in the scientific method of nursing that is based on a strong foundation of knowledge and skill. This method is used to gather and evaluate information about a patient so that an intelligent plan of care can be identified. Levine views a diagnosis as predictive, statistical, and essential for medicine. She believes nurses should develop testable hypotheses or assumptions in order to provide valid nursing intervention. Basic to gathering data are the vital observations made by the nurse in relation to a unique individual. Observation must be relevant, continuously made over time to consider changing conditions, and based on the expected outcome. Untoward or unexpected responses may demand immediate attention. The nursing process can be utilized with Levine's theory as shown in Table 7-7.

Table 7-7

Levine Nursing Process

Nursing Process	Scientific Method	Nursing Implications	Examples
Assessment	Assess unique needs based on knowledge and skills. Continuously gather relevant information in relation to a changing condition	Gather data based on the individual's integrated response arising from the internal environment. Identify the level of energy, the ability to heal after a loss of structural integrity, and then the personal and social integrity, including level of independence, relationship with family, and decision-making ability.	The patient was admitted two days ago, has burns over her hands, and is unable to hold a glass of water. She feels helpless and complains about being isolated from her family because she is in the hospital. Her dressings are removed daily, and the burned area is healing.
Diagnosis	Develop assumptions/hypotheses about the four conservation areas.	Base assumptions on holistic concerns that reflect the uniqueness of the individual.	First and second degree burns of both hands causes a deficit in ability to perform self-care activities independently. Social isolation related to separation from family members.

Plan	Identify nursing interventions that are therapeutic or supportive of adaptation on the part of the patient.	Plans should reflect and test out assumptions about the projected outcome of care in all four areas of conservation.	Contact family to visit the patient. Provide utensils that will facilitate independence. Allow the patient to rest so that her energy is not wasted. Monitor condition of dressings. Communicate with the patient about the effects of the burns and about the healing process. Provide privacy during family visits. Provide a straw so that patient can drink without assistance. Assist the physician in changing dressings.
Implementation	Focus on the interaction/communication of the nurse and patient while performing nursing measures. Continue to observe for change.	The nurse must be attentive and prompt in meeting needs. Communicate both socially and as a teacher.	
Evaluation	Continually observe the effect of intervention on the patient's progress related to level of adaptation.	Evaluation is viewed as a constant activity.	Measure the patient's level of energy, her ability to drink without help, and assess the degree of healing and her interaction with her family.

Incorporated into the nursing process are the major concepts of the theory as incorporated into the model. The nurse and patient communicated about the healing process (structural integrity), privacy was provided to reduce the sense of isolation (social integrity), a straw was provided to increase the patient's independence (personal integrity), and efforts were made to conserve the patient's energy.

Evaluation

The major focus of the theory—the *interactive process* between the patient and the nurse and between the internal and external environment—is not developed sufficiently to be clearly understood. Aside from the recognition that individuals are unique, and need to feel safe and to have their needs met promptly, there is little specific guidance as to what is characteristic of a positive communication. The relationship between the major concepts of the four areas of conservation is also unclear, even though the theory supports the holistic approach. Levine uses the words *wholistic* and *holistic* interchangeably, as do other theorists, but Levine prefers *holistic* since it tends to connote a greater sense of "entire" structural integrity as it relates to anatomy and physiology. The concept *energy,* aside from the simplistic definition of *work,* is very abstract, especially as related to *holistic.* There is a notion of energy that is used during the disease process and returned after rest. Levine characterizes both the conservation areas of *personal* and *social integrity* by the use of abstract concepts that are not defined. If one is to use the scientific method and develop hypotheses, all these concepts would have to be clearer. One nurse's assessment of a patient's sense of identity or self-image could be quite different from another nurse's assessment. Thus the major concepts and their relationships are, for the most part, abstract and unclear.

Because there is no model provided with this theory, and because there is a lack of clarity between the concepts, the development of a model must be based on inferred assumptions, which could lead to a misinterpretation of the theory. Again, multiple interpretations of assumptions could lead to much confusion in nursing practice.

The concept of the *environment* has the greatest clarity. Much of Levine's writing centers around the internal environment, such as the failure of the nervous system, the hormonal system, fluid and electrolyte balance, and nutritional, oxygen, and growth needs. Cellular growth and the inflammatory process are also reviewed in detail. This emphasis supports a greater understanding of the medical approach to patient care, which is basically empirical and inferential in its approach to concepts. The *external environment* is reviewed with some clarity, and the concept provides a way of viewing patients more holistically in terms of the forces that affect their behaviors.

The concept of *adaptation,* although it is the goal of care and is related to a state of health, is not clearly defined; one can draw the assumption that with healing and structural integrity, adaptation can occur. Basic to that idea is the notion that one's self-image or family relationships are altered as a result of the illness experience and return to "normal" after the patient leaves the hospital.

JOYCE TRAVELBEE: DESCRIPTION OF THE THEORY

Central to Travelbee's theory is the *interpersonal process,* which is viewed as a human-to-human relationship that forms during an experience of suffering. Thus, an understanding of the concepts *human, illness,* and *suffering* is essential in order to incorporate the concepts into a process. *Humans* refer to both the individual who is ill and the nurse who provides an intellectual approach to nursing care.

Model

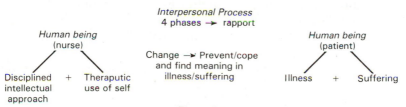

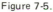

Figure 7-5.

The model is reflective of Travelbee's major concepts and the relationship among them. The following propositions can be drawn from the model:

1. Human beings engage in an interpersonal process.
2. Nursing involves a disciplined intellectual approach and the therapeutic use of self.
3. Human beings (patients) experience illness and suffering.
4. The interpersonal process has four phases, with the goal of establishing rapport.
5. Involved in the interpersonal process is change, which enables the patient to prevent, cope with, and find meaning in illness and suffering.

These propositions form the basis of the theory which guides the nurse not only to deal with illness but also to promote health in the care of individuals, families, and communities. Note that the concept of the *environment* is very limited and relates mostly to the hospital, where the ill individual is found.

Travelbee makes some philosophical assumptions about *human beings*. The following represent the highlights of a few:

1. Human beings are irreplaceable and unique.
2. As biological organisms, they are affected, influenced, and changed by heredity, environment, culture, and life experiences.
3. Individuals can go beyond the material aspects of their world, which is both limited and unlimited.
4. Humans experience conflict and make choices.
5. Human beings are capable of rational, logical thinking, and maturity.
6. Although individuals possess a sense of aloneness that is elusive, they also possess the ability to feel understood.
7. As social beings, they are able to know, love, and respond to the uniqueness of others.
8. Human beings strive to rise above their limitations and above such human conditions as loneliness, restlessness, and dissatisfaction.
9. Humans recognize that they will die, and death remains abstract.
10. Humans have the capacity to evolve and change over time.

Key to the assumptions about human beings is that in order to understand them, one must search out their uniqueness. Individuals are affected by their environments, their previous choices, their relationships with others, and their own understanding of death. Thus, the human experience of illness and suffering must be viewed from the unique perspective of the individual.

Travelbee has also developed certain assumptions about illness and suffering. The following relate to illness:

1. During illness one rearranges one's priorities.
2. Illness reminds one of how frail human beings actually are.
3. To be ill is to be lonely and to realize how minimally others can grasp the meaning of illness.
4. Fear of the known and unknown is profound in terms of one's ability to cope during illness.

5. Illness creates worries about economics, dependents, ability to adapt, pain, and fatigue.
6. Illness increases a sense of loneliness and helplessness, and a fear of death.
7. Illness changes one's ability to sleep and to handle the frustration created by small events and pain.

Suffering, which involves discomfort and anguish, is experienced during illness by the individual and his loved ones. Suffering relates to the following:

1. feelings of intense pain, both physical and emotional
2. waiting for a loved one to visit
3. learning that a loved one has a fatal illness and not sharing that knowledge
4. feelings of overwhelming stress and tiredness.

The integration of the assumptions about human beings, illness, and suffering leads one to understand why Travelbee emphasizes the interpersonal relationship between humans. The labels *nurse* and *patient* are viewed as supporting the stereotypes found in literature.

The concept *nurse* is viewed from the perspective of both the characteristics of human beings and the role of the nurse in the interpersonal process. Involved in nursing is the ability to bring about change while assisting individuals, families, and the community. Most of the theory focuses on a human-to-human relationship, so the nurse assists the family and the community by helping and focusing on individuals. There seems little emphasis on group process.

The nurse's role is viewed in relation to *health*. Nursing's goal is to help individuals prevent illness and suffering and maintain the highest possible level of health. Health is seen as *subjective,* defined by the individual's perception, and *objective*, involving the absence of discernable disease, disability, or defect as assessed by a spiritual director or psychological counselor. The subjective and objective appraisals of the individual's health status can differ. Travelbee supports the increasing emphasis on health promotion and disability prevention. Health teaching helps individuals to find meaning in illness and provides measures to maintain health; it is not just the imparting of information.

Professional nurses use a disciplined intellectual approach to care, which involves a logical method of approaching problems, the knowledge and understanding of concepts and principles, and the ability to use the knowledge in caring for others. Key to logical thinking is reflecting, reasoning, and deliberating, which should lead to creative and intelligent actions. The nurse's therapeutic use of self requires insight, self-understanding, an understanding of human behavior, and the ability to intervene effectively. The use of intuition or hit-or-miss methods of care are inappropriate. Compassion and empathy are appropriate emotions when the nurse also has insight. Commitment to and confirmation of one's responsibility as a nurse are essential.

The human-to-human relationship and its components, the four interlocking phases that lead to rapport, are basic to the theory (see Table 7-8). The initial judgments are made by the nurse during the *original encounter*. The focus and goal during this phase are to see the patient as a unique human being rather than as a stereotype. When that is accomplished, the phase of *emerging identities* begins, as both human beings begin to establish a bond based on their similarities and differences. At that point, *empathy* is felt on a conscious level, and the ability to predict behavior increases. *Sympathy* occurs when there is a desire to alleviate the distress, and actions can occur. The goal of *rapport* follows, which provides a relationship in which suffering can be reduced or minimized. These phases reflect a positive maturing approach to human relationships. Relationships that tend to stereotype patients, involve superficial interactions, and are based on a lack of awareness of one's own feelings tend to alienate the patient and do not lead to rapport. The assumption is that such a negative relationship is limited in its ability to alleviate suffering and assist the patient in coping with illness.

A major assumption which strongly affects the human-to-human relationship is that effective communication must take place. Communication, *which is verbal and nonverbal,* is a reciprocal dynamic process by which meanings are exchanged between individuals. Verbal communication uses written and spoken words. Nonverbal communication involves gestures, facial expressions, and body movements. Crying, groaning, and screaming communicate feelings. Nonverbal communication is continuous, and the sensitivity and receptiveness of the receiver will affect his ability to sense or perceive the sender's intentions. The goal of communication is to understand *what* is to be accomplished in the interaction, *why* the events are occurring, and *how* to achieve the goal. Involved in such communication is observation, which is necessary for data collection so that inferences can be made.

Communication techniques that facilitate the goal of establishment of rapport and reduction of suffering should be used. Any technique that achieves those goals is appropriate. Offering open-ended

Table 7-8

Travelbee's Human-to-Human Relationship Model

| | Verbal and Nonverbal Communication | | | |
| | | Interlocking Phases | | |
Original Encounter →	Emerging Identities →	Empathy →	Sympathy →	Rapport →
Development of initial judgments	Ability to appreciate the other's uniqueness	Shared psychological states	Desire to alleviate distress	Process by which two individuals perceive and behave toward each other in a positive manner
Positive relationship Observation to develop inferences Emerges from a stereotyping approach to the recognition of the uniqueness of the ill person	Establishment of a bond based on the uniqueness of human beings Similarities and dissimilarities emerge with understanding	Neutral process: nonaction Can see beyond outward behavior Conscious process Focus on similarities Leads to the ability to predict behavior An awareness of value judgment	Action oriented (absent in empathy) Involved with and comprehends the distress of others and feels compassion Relieves others from feeling alone	Stereotypes are removed There are moments of relatedness, and a freeing of energy Increases confidence of ill persons in those who care for them Dynamic, with varying degrees and levels
Negative relationship View human as stereotyped patient Develop snap judgments Interact superficially and mechanically Inability to recognize human differences	Overidentification with patient: cannot separate nurse problem from patient problem Transient feelings of envy Lack of interest in other person	Identification, in which one strives to be like the other, and projection, in which one attributes one's own tendencies to another function without awareness	Objective detachment and alienation Objectifying pity in a dehumanizing way: humans are perceived as objects	No rapport established There is nurse-patient distance

comments that support reflective techniques and sharing perceptions facilitate communication, while using clichés discourages it. Communication breaks down when there is failure to perceive the ill person as a human being, failure to recognize the real rather than the surface meaning of communication, failure to listen, tendency to accuse and blame, and to use value statements without reflection. The guiding principle for the nurse is that she should explore with the ill person any comment that she does not understand.

Application to the Nursing Process

The purpose of nursing is to meet the nursing needs of the individual and family by assisting them to prevent or cope with the experience of illness and suffering. Travelbee identifies five steps which guide the nurse in determining and planning care. These steps must

Table 7-9

Nursing Process	Travelbee's Steps in Meeting Nursing Needs	Implications
Assessment	Make systematic observations and develop inferences as to the nature of the need, and validate these with the ill individual	(The individual is experiencing surgery) Assess cognitive clarity—the individual's comprehension of what is happening Assess anxiety level related to such things as the meaning of the affected body organ or part to the individual, and fear of pain and disfigurement
Diagnosis	Formulate a need-oriented diagnosis Identify need for referral if necessary	Anxiety Need for information Need to explore surgical experience and illness
Plan	Identify learning needs Decide the method by which the need can be met Determine when the need should be met Identify alternative ways of meeting the needs	Build security in relation to the individual's need to believe that he will survive surgery Continually explore what the ill individual feels and understands Relate meaning of illness to the individual
Implementation	Meet needs through the interpersonal process	Provide information and meet needs that relate to suffering. Listen, develop, and validate inference made
Evaluation	Identify changes in the individual's behavior, and explore whether needs have been met	Note level of anxiety throughout surgical experience.

be used in conjunction with the four interlocking phases of the interpersonal process and can be compared to the steps of the nursing process, as shown in Table 7-9.

Although it is somewhat difficult to identify from the approach described, the major emphasis of this theory is on human relationships. In the assessment phase, assuming that rapport has been established, the nurse makes observations that lead to inferences. This is quite different from approaching a patient with the expectation of the "typical" patient reaction to surgery and providing only a limited amount of information. When the four phases are used, the following is likely to occur: During the *original encounter*, stereotyping is reduced, and the nurse sees the ill individual as a unique person who is experiencing surgery. Information is shared by the nurse, who allows the ill person to reflect on the meaning of that information. Previous life experiences are discussed as they relate to the present situation. This communication leads to a bonding relationship as *identities emerge. Empathy* evolves when the nurse can see and understand the real meaning of the surgical experience to the individual. This "real" meaning is expressed verbally by spoken words and nonverbally by physiological signs such as anorexia, insomnia, fatigue, and headache. *Sympathy* follows as anxiety is discussed and the desire to reduce the anxiety level emerges. When *rapport* has been established in the relationship, nursing implementation can occur that will ultimately reduce the anxiety and suffering (see Table 7-8).

Evaluation

The major concepts within the theory are well defined in Travelbee's writings. *Human suffering* and *interpersonal process* have definite characteristics, which add clarity. Nursing concepts that are not clearly defined are the *environment, community,* and the *family.* Since the major focus of the theory is on *illness,* the characteristics of *health* are rather abstract. *Illness* is more reflective of the physiological aspects of the human being. The psychosocial-spiritual aspects of the human condition are discussed as they relate to illness and suffering.

The interlocking phases of the interpersonal process basically flow from one to the other, so that a significant therapeutic relationship can develop. It is not clear whether all the phases consistently occur depending on the specific communication, or if once rapport has been established, the phases are not significant: Probably the truth is somewhere in the middle.

The theory is descriptive in nature and is not too difficult to understand if one accepts the fact that nursing, as a profession, is more abstract than empirical.

JEAN WATSON:
DESCRIPTION OF THE THEORY

In describing her "philosophy and science of caring," Watson provides basic assumptions about the science of caring in nursing: Caring is an interpersonal process composed of carative factors that result in the meeting of human needs. Caring promotes health, accepts persons as they are or may become, and creates an environment that allows persons to choose the best actions for themselves. Thus, the major concepts of the theory are *caring, interpersonal, needs,* and *growth.* Decision making is the individual's responsibility. Nursing intervention is based on a scientific-humanistic approach from a carative viewpoint.

Watson identifies ten primary carative factors that form the basis for studying and understanding nursing as a science of caring (see Table 7-10). The first three are the philosophical foundations for the science. The others, except the last, have more of a scientific data base. The last is quite philosophical and relates to understanding people from the standpoint of their perceptions of life experiences such as pain and death.

Table 7-10

Carative Factors

Factors	Components and Implications
Humanistic-altruistic system of values	Humanism involves kindness, concern for, and love of self and others.
	Altruism requires appreciation of diversity and individuality.
	Development of a value system necessitates exploration of different philosophies, beliefs, and life-styles.
	A value system provides a foundation for empathy, promotes maturity, satisfaction, and integrity, and develops an extension of the self.
Instillation of faith and hope	Faith and hope help the patient to accept information, change attitudes, and develop health-seeking behaviors.
	Instilling hope requires the discovery of what is meaningful and important to the individual.
	In instilling faith and hope, one goes beyond the limitations of the scientific approach and uses the belief in the healing power, which supports the holistic approach.

Table 7-10 (*cont.*)

Factors	Components and Implications
Cultivation of sensitivity to oneself and to others	Sensitivity encourages the recognition of feelings. Sensitivity to oneself relates to self-actualization through self-acceptance and psychological growth. Honesty toward the self promotes authenticity and sensitivity toward others. The patient and nurse retain their own separate identities.
Development of a helping/trust relationship	In a trust relationship, there is greater potential for promoting psychological and social growth and development and for facilitating health-seeking behaviors. A trust relationship is critical in order to establish rapport. The nurse must get to know the other person's self, life space, and what affects, motivates, or inhibits health-seeking behavior. Genuineness is brought to the relationship through honesty and authenticity, which minimizes the playing of roles. Empathy is experienced, which reflects the ability of the nurse to experience the other person's private world and feelings without discomfort, fear, anger, or conflict. Nonpossessive warmth promotes the other person's growth. Communication involves the *somatic* level (the bio-physiological states), the *action* level (movement and gait), and the *language* level (words and their meaning.) Communications have personal meaning to individual's; thus validation is essential.
Promotion and acceptance of the expression of positive and negative feelings.	Acceptance of feelings is part of the development of a helping/trust relationship. Inconsistency between thoughts and feelings can lead to anxiety, stress, confusion, or fear. Cognitive and affective factors affect feelings that need to be expressed in strong emotional statements.
Systematic use of the scientific problem-solving method for decision making	The nursing process and the scientific process are basically the same. Without the scientific method, the nurse uses tenacity by holding on to old ideas, intuition by knowing before the facts, and authority which is seen as law.
Promotion of interpersonal teaching-learning	Health teaching is one of the major functions of nursing. Information promotes accurate expectation and reduces discomfort. Information increases one's ability to predict and feel more in control.

Table 7-10 (cont.)

Factors	Components and Implications
	Information can change beliefs and reduce fantasies.
	Information involves the evaluation of threatening situations and ways of reducing threats.
Provision of a supportive, protective, and/or corrective mental, physical, sociocultural, and spiritual environment	Interdependence exists between the external and internal environments which influence health and illness.
	Stress results from and includes anything that interrupts planned activities, and can cause illness.
	Comfort can come from the external environment of the hospital, which is usually viewed as stressful.
	Privacy serves to maintain human dignity and integrity.
	Anxiety involves a clean, aesthetic environment in which potential hazards have been eliminated.
Assistance with the gratification of needs	A need is a requirement of a person that, if supported, relieves immediate distress and improves the sense of adequacy and well-being. There are *lower order needs,* which are biophysical and necessary for survival (such as food), and psychophysical needs, which are functional needs (such as activity); and *higher order needs,* which are psychosocial and integrative (such as achievement), and intra- and interpersonal needs, which are growth seeking.
Allowance for existential/ phenomenological force	Allowing for existential forces acknowledges the separateness and identity of each person, and gives personal meaning to the human predicament.
	An existential philosophy enables the nurse to approach things from a holistic framework in order to understand the individuality of persons and to understand the way they see things.
	Individuals can feel understood in a world that is unfair at times.
	Existentialism recognizes that there is no escape from pain, death, or ultimate aloneness, or from one's own responsibility for the way one's life is lived.

Model

Within the interpretive model shown in Figure 7-6 the basic concepts are identified within each of the carative factors, as is the goal of enabling the individual to experience a positive health change. The model is both foundational and linear. The first three factors are within a box, since they are integrated and interdependent. The possession of *values* and the ability to extend oneself altruistically are closely linked to one's ability to approach persons in a *positive* manner from the somewhat nontraditional approach of holistic healing

Interpretation of Watson's Model

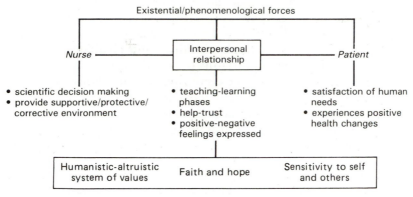

Figure 7-6.

through *faith* and *hope*. Watson believes that without these concepts, an interpersonal relationship involving *teaching and learning, help and trust,* and the *acceptance of feelings* would not be possible. These factors describe the human characteristics essential for the nurse and the individual who is ill.

Humans also have needs that are described similarly to those developed by Maslow (see Chapter 5). The lower-order needs are both biophysical (food/fluid) and psychophysical (activity/sexuality), and the higher-order needs are psychosocial (affiliation/achievement) and interpersonal (self-actualization). The highest need is for interpersonal relationships, which is the basis of the theory and the most significant activity in the science of caring. *Curing* is viewed very differently and is reflective of the domain of medicine.

The concept *environment* refers to a caring climate in which the individual can develop his potential by choosing what is best for him at any given point in time. It also describes the *internal environment* as related to biophysical human needs, and the *external environment,* which includes stress, change, comfort, privacy, and safety. *Stress* is viewed as anything that interrupts usual or planned life activities. These interruptions involve cultural, social, or interpersonal changes that may cause a change in health. The hospital environment, in which the individual loses his identity and independence, and which is inflexible and bound by tradition, creates a lack of comfort and privacy. Privacy supports personal autonomy and emotional release and helps in self-evaluation. A safe environment relates to the prevention of accidents as well as the use of immunizations.

Health is a process of adapting, coping, and growing throughout life, and includes a balanced life, a sense of happiness, and the ability to change. The absence of illness, a high level of overall physical, mental, and social functioning, and a general adaptative maintenance level also connote a health state. Health relates to stress-linked illnesses, developmental conflicts, and loss. Each phase of growth and development brings certain vulnerabilities and challenges that can be stressful. Loss is a highly variable personal experience, such as loss related to body image, and occurs during each developmental period.

Nursing is viewed as an interpersonal caring process. The nursing process is similar to the research process, which leads to scientific decision making. Review the following and note the similarities in the processes:

Nursing Process	Research Process	Watson's Nursing Process

Assessment	Formulate problem
	Review literature
	Formulate theoretical
	    framework
		Involve observations, use of
		    knowledge, and a theoretical
		    framework

Diagnosis	Formulate hypothesis (some-
	    thing assumed)
		Formulate a problem-oriented
		    hypothesis

Plan	Define variables (something
	    that varies/changes)
		Review variables
		Design care based on framework
		Determine further data to be
		    collected

Implementation	Obtain/collect data	Direct action and implement a plan

Evaluation	Analyze and evaluate data
	Determine results
	Communicate results
		Review method of analyzing
		    data and the effects of
		    implementation
		Interpret results of care

All these processes provide a way of thinking about nursing from a scientific, problem-solving perspective. In research, the goal, which is long range, is to learn something new and increase the body of knowledge. In nursing, the goal is more immediate and refers to assisting an ill individual to become healthier by using the existing body of nursing knowledge to enhance understanding of a holistic person. The nursing process also focuses on the empirical or concrete more than does the research process, which may lead to more abstract findings.

Incorporated into the nursing process are seven clinical care phases that are reflective of interpersonal *teaching-learning* processes and that can be used for both healthy and ill persons. The nurse (1) *scans* in order to describe the person's goals or problems based on his own perception, (2) *formulates* the problem while receiving feedback through words, gestures, and so on, (3) *appraises* the problem jointly with the individual and identifies its significance, (4) shares the need for *problem solving* with the individual, (5) jointly *plans* strategies and techniques to use, (6) *implements* care by providing cognitive information, and (7) *evaluates* whether or not the preparation or teaching has helped the person learn or cope. These phases of care must incorporate the curative factors, especially those that most relate to the caring relationship, to be effective.

Application to the Nursing Process

During the *assessment* phase, it is important for the nurse to identify the individual's *phenomenal field,* which reflects both the person's self within his life space and the factors that motivate or inhibit his health-seeking behaviors. Data must be obtained in relation to his need for information and ability to solve problems and deal with stress and change, developmental conflicts, losses, and needs.

The *diagnosis,* which results from the analysis of the data and the development of assumptions (which Watson calls *hypotheses*), relates to the individual's state of health and ability to cope, adapt, grow developmentally, and deal with loss.

The *plan* provides multiple alternatives, using the problem-solving approach, by which human needs can be met. The individual works with the nurse to formulate strategies and techniques that will be useful to him.

Implementation includes reinforcing the individual's faith and hope so that attitudes and health-seeking behaviors can change. Interpersonal communication involves genuineness, openness, honesty, nonpossessiveness, and warmth. Privacy is provided and the environment is one that is supportive and protective.

Evaluation reviews whether health-seeking behaviors have emerged and whether the individual's needs have been met.

Although there are no specific phases provided during the interpersonal process, except the seven clinical care phases during the teaching-learning process, one can assume that the theory incorporates all its concepts into every communication between the nurse and the client. These concepts, such as honesty, trust, and openness, are very abstract and require a period of time to develop between two human beings. Thus, phases do occur as sharing and trust increase with time.

Evaluation

Watson's theory is descriptive and explains the nurse-patient structure from both theoretical and philosophical frameworks. The concepts, such as those described under the category of biophysical needs, like oxygen and food, are basically empirical and are often measured by inference; yet the vast majority of the concepts, such as caring, self-esteem, and trust, are abstract and, although defined by Watson, remain unclear in their definitions. For example, *empathy* is defined as the nurse's ability to experience the other person's private world and feelings. How does one measure whether one has entered the private world of another when perceptions tend to differ substantially? Considering the fact that the nurse and the patient have different life experiences and needs, can feelings be clearly shared and mutually felt? These abstract concepts need continued definition and further development of characteristics that specifically relate to each.

The theory incorporates concepts from *basic needs* to *existentialism*. One must have a sound foundation in the natural and behavioral sciences and in philosophical and logical thought processes in order to use the theory in nursing practice. Thus, whether the theory is simple or complex is based on one's educational and experiential background. There is nothing contradictory within the theory, nor does it negate existing knowledge.

This theory, with its emphasis on the relationship between the nurse and the ill individual, has been categorized as an interaction theory. It does focus on human needs and utilizes Maslow's hierarchy, however, and could also have been identified as a need theory. Because the major concepts are so abstract and deal almost exclusively with the significance of the caring relationship, though, it seems more appropriate for this section of the book. In addition, Watson is not need oriented in isolation, but only from the framework of meeting human needs through the interpersonal caring relationship.

SUMMARY
OF INTERACTION THEORIES

As noted in Table 7-11, the interaction theories have as their major focus the relationship between the counselor and the client or nurse and the individual who is ill or has a felt need. All the interaction theories focus on a supportive, therapeutic interaction. The degree of

Table 7-11

Carl Rogers's Theory
and Selected Interaction-Oriented Nursing Theories

Theorist	Role of Counselor/Nurse	Focus
Carl Rogers	The counselor assumes the client's internal frame of reference through empathic understanding. Behavior must be understood from the internal frame of reference of the individual himself.	In effective therapy that uses the nondirective approach, there is a decrease in psychological *tension.* During the latter part of the change process, the client increasingly discusses plans and behavioral steps.
Peplau	Counseling facilitates self-directed actions and deals with how a person feels about what is happening. The therapeutic process gives further direction to the individual's growth and maturational development.	Individuals seek assistance based on a felt *need,* with the goal of reducing tension. There are four interlocking phases of the nurse-patient relationship. As old needs are met, the individual is free for more productive activities and relationships.
Hall	The nurse uses reflective techniques, acting as a mirror for the patient to explore feelings.	The individual explores and uncovers his difficulty, *problem,* or *threat.* Individuals realize their motivation and grow in self-awareness, which helps them to cope with and face the future.
Levine	Nurses use human interaction with supportive and therapeutic interventions in relation to the four conservation principles.	Changes in the individual's level of adaptation and maintenance of the integrity are emphasized. Verbal and nonverbal communication are an integral part of the interpersonal process.
Travelbee	Nursing, a disciplined intellectual approach, uses the self therapeutically in relation to illness and suffering and their meaning to the patient.	The human-to-human interaction has four interlocking phases that lead to rapport, which helps individuals to prevent or cope with and find meaning in illness and suffering.
Watson	The nurse provides a supportive, protective, curative environment incorporating a humanistic-altruistic interpersonal system that includes faith, hope, and trust.	Humanistic values and altruistic behavior are used with consciousness raising about one's views, beliefs, and values in relation to human needs. Uses carative factors with a scientific problem-solving process while incorporating phenomenology and existential thinking in order to deal with developmental conflicts and needs, and changes in health behavior.

clarity of descriptions of what specifically occurs during the interpersonal/interactive phases of the relationship differs from theory to theory. Levine relates mostly to the purposes of the interaction rather than to the specific details of the encounter. Hall provides a framework that is very abstract—the notion of a mirror to explore feelings—but does not clearly explain how one proceeds to practice within that framework. Carl Rogers, Peplau, and Travelbee provide similar ideas on what the interactive process really includes, and thus their theories are more functional. Rogers's *experiences of exploration* are rather similar to Peplau's *orientation phase* and Travelbee's *four phases* that lead to *rapport*.

Needs are stressed in Watson's theory, mentioned in Peplau's, and implied in Hall's and Levine's. The concept of *maturity, growth,* and *development* is strong in Peplau's and Watson's theories. All the nursing theories are supportive of Carl Rogers's nondirective approach to helping individuals with some sort of psychological tension.

The following common assumptions can be drawn from the interaction theories:

1. The relationship between the client or patient and the nurse or counselor has a significant impact on the client's/patient's ability to deal with needs and to cope.
2. The individual's internal frame of reference must be the focus of both verbal and nonverbal communication.
3. The counselor or nurse acts as a facilitator of human development.
4. In dealing with individuals in an interactive way, concepts such as *self-awareness* and *tension,* although abstract, are useful as a focus.

Within all these theories (except perhaps Watson's) the concepts of the *environment* and *health* and their meanings to the interpersonal process are limited. In the systems theories, on the other hand, the individual and his relationship with the environment is the major emphasis. Interaction theories, like need theories, focus on the characteristics of human beings and the role of the nurse.

REFERENCES

Bates, M. "Naturalist at Large" *Natural History* (June/July 1967) 76:10.

Hall, L.E. "Another View of Nursing Care and Quality." In *Continu-*

ity of Patient Care: The Role of Nursing, edited by K.M. Straub and K.S. Parker, pp. 47-60. Washington, D.C.: Catholic University Press, 1966.

Levine, M.E. *Introduction to Clinical Nursing,* 2d ed. Philadelphia: F.A. Davis Company, 1973.

Peplau, H.E. *Interpersonal Relations in Nursing.* New York: G.P. Putnam's Sons, 1952.

Rogers, C. *Counseling and Psychotherapy: Newer Concepts in Practice.* Boston: Houghton Mifflin Company, 1942.

Rogers, C. *Client Centered Therapy; its Current Practice, Implications and Theory.* Boston: Houghton Mifflin Company, 1951.

Travelbee, J. *Interpersonal Aspects of Nursing,* 2d ed. Philadelphia: F.A. Davis Company, 1971.

Watson, J. *Nursing: The Philosophy and Science of Caring.* Boston: Little, Brown & Company, 1979.

8

INTEGRATION OF NURSING THEORIES

INTRODUCTION

At this point in the history of nursing theory, it is relatively safe to identify four major themes that have evolved. Although none of them has clear-cut distinctions from the others, they present sufficient differences in their approaches to the major concepts and to the nursing process to warrant separate identifications. For example, Hall emphasizes the *core*—nondirective counseling that facilitates the patients' understanding of themselves—yet recognizes the caring aspects in relation to meeting patient needs. She is also quite concerned with the effects of the hospital environment on the patient. Thus, Hall's theory has an emphasis that is within the framework of the interaction theme as well as the environmental and need themes. Yet in reviewing some of the theories, such as Henderson's, the need theme is clearly appropriate and obvious. Peplau's theory can be viewed only within the interaction theme. The placement of a particular theory within the framework of a particular theme has served mostly for comparison.

Among the themes there are different major focuses (see Table 8-1). All themes focus on the human being, mostly as an individual. The individual is universally described as being ill or well, experiencing changes, having needs, capable of interacting with the environment and with others, and being relatively unique, although with common growth and development characteristics. Both the need theories and interaction theories are particularly oriented toward describing the role of the nurse in terms of these characteristics. The environment's impact on the human being is focused upon in the environmental and systems theories. Their difference basically relates to either the immediate physical environment or an open-systems environment that is all-inclusive of humans and the forces that affect them. It should be noted that none of the theorists or themes emphasizes health as a major focus except to view it as a state or condition of the human being. Thus, it is the most peripheral of the concepts and relates primarily to the goal of nursing care.

FOUNDATION FOR THE USE OF NURSING THEORY

In reviewing the theories, it becomes evident that an understanding of certain arts and sciences enhances understanding of the theories. The most significant of these are anatomy, physiology, pathophysiology, and psychology. Other disciplines, such as sociology, philosophy, and religion, are also important but are more peripheral to the essence of the theories. Many theorists mention the family and the community—which, as groups, are related to sociology—but do not significantly deal with other kinds of groups.

The focus of the theories is on the individual and the nurse. From anatomy and physiology comes an understanding of the basic physical needs that seem to be a primary focus in almost all the need theories. Pathophysiology is particularly important, because most of the theories deal with the ill person. Orem, for example, emphasizes self-care deficits related to needs evolving from health deviation states, Orlando focuses on the immediate needs of the patient who is ill, and Johnson recognizes that stress affects certain subsystems, causing instability.

Psychological theories such as Maslow's and Murray's need theories, Parson's system theory, and Erickson's developmental theories offer a strong base of knowledge in the understanding of nursing theories. Freud and Carl Rogers also had a real impact on the interaction theories. Hans Selye's writing on stress theory has influenced nurse theorists and provides a framework through which to understand Betty Neuman's theory.

It would probably be impossible to understand nursing theories

Table 8-1
Integrating Major Concepts
with Theoretical Themes

Major Nursing Concepts	Environment	Need	System	Interaction
Major Focus	Humans/Environment	Humans/Nursing	Humans/Environment	Humans/Nurse
Humans	Humans are affected by their physical, emotional, and social environment.	Humans are sick or well and have physical, emotional, and social needs.	The human is a unified whole within an open system, and has pattern, organization, and perceptions that influence the behavior system.	Humans are capable of engaging in an interactive process and experience conflict, developmental crisis, and illness, and have needs.
Environment	The environment is all things that are external to the patient and that influence the reparative process.	The environment affects human development and the achievement of needs.	The environment affects humans, who are part of the environment, through forces, stress, energy, information, and stimuli.	The environment is based on the perception of the individual and is basically external in the forrm of stress and stimuli.
Health	*Health* is the absence of disease which is a reparative process.	Health relates to sustaining life processes, and maintaining integrating function, a state of adequacy, and self-direction in meeting human needs.	Health is the ability to maintain integration, balance, and maximum potential through effective adaptation, goal setting, and reconstitution.	Health is a process of full growth and development and adaptation, and is the goal when illness or a perceived need occurs.
Nursing	*Nursing* is a way of facilitating nature's reparative process by placing patients in the condition for nature to act upon them.	Nursing assists patients in meeting their needs and helping themselves whenever possible.	Nursing is oriented toward the individual to respond to the variables within the environment in a positive manner.	Nursing is an interpersonal humanistic process involving verbal and nonverbal communication and mutual exploration of feelings and perceptions.

without some basic background in pure and behavioral sciences. Reviewing the nursing theories should encourage learners to return to their science books for greater clarity and understanding.

AN INTEGRATED MODEL

There are certain inevitabilities in the development of an integrated model. It will *not* adequately represent any one theorist or group of theorists because all their major concepts would not be included. The relationship between the concepts would *not* comprehensively reflect of any of the major themes. In essence, it is unlikely that any of the theorists could support such a model in total. Nevertheless, the model in Figure 8-1 is developed so that readers can use it as a starting point in creating their own.

Integrated Model from Nursing Theories

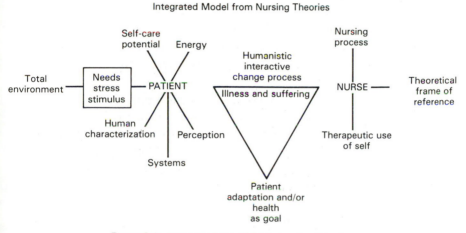

Figure 8-1. Integrated model from nursing theories.

The concepts within the model are basically abstract; thus the following definitions are provided to increase clarity.

Definition of Terms

Patient—Nursing Care Recipient

Energy—natural power, and the capacity to act and be active, such as to do work

Human characteristics—attributes that make and distinguish an individual; contain both unique and representative features

Perception—an individual's mental image of the environment based on cognition and experience

Self-care potential—level of ability to provide for own needs independently

System—interacting, interdependent forces of the personal, interpersonal, and social aspects of individuals and groups that also have subsystems, patterns, and organization

Environment— Surrounding Conditions

Need—a lack of something requisite, desirable, or useful; or a physiological or psychological requirement for the well-being of an organism

Stimulus—something that causes activity

Stress—physical, chemical, or emotional force that causes bodily or mental tension

Nurse—Care Provider

Nursing process—a systematic and analytical approach designed to change the patient's situation toward the achievement of specific goals

Theoretical frame of reference—a structural way of viewing a nurse-patient situation by the systematic use of concepts and propositions that describe, explain, or predict practice

Therapeutic use of self—the use of self-understanding; ability to interpret one's behavior with intellect, reasoning, and compassion in order to facilitate the goal of nursing.

Health— Goal of Patient-Nurse
Interaction

Adaptation—change process of adjusting and responding to the total environment

Health—state in which the holistic individual sustains life processes through integration and balance and functions at an optimum level of well-being

Interactive Process—Link between Patient
and Nurse

Change process—an approach to care in which there is conscious utilization and application of knowledge as an instrument for modifying patterns of holistic behavior

Humanistic—an approach, attitude, or way of functioning that centers around human interests and values; a philosophy that asserts the dignity and worth of humans and their capacity for self-realization

Illness—an unhealthy condition of a holistic individual

Suffering—involving distress, pain, or death

There are certain relationships that should be noted within the integrated model (Fig. 8-1). The one basic and primary relationship is that the *environment* affects the *patient* and that the patient and *nurse* interact in relation to *health*. Note that the four major concepts in nursing are included. Other relationships include the following:

The patient and the nurse relate through a humanistic interactive change process during illness and suffering.

The patient and the nurse attempt to achieve the goal of patient adaptation and/or health.

The total environment affects the needs, stress, and stimulus of the patient.

The nursing process, theoretical frame of reference, and the therapeutic use of self relate to the nurse.

Human characteristics, systems, perception, self-care potential, and energy relate to the patient.

One can identify the major concepts from a variety of theorists within this model, especially when the definitions are included. Note Nightingale's *environment,* Peplau's and Watson's *humanistic interactive interpersonal process* and the *therapeutic use of self,* Henderson's *needs,* Levine's and Rogers's *energy approach,* Orem's *self-care potential,* King's *perception* and *systems,* Roy's *stimulus* and *adaptation,* and Travelbee's approach to *suffering* and *illness. Health* as a goal is reflective of all the theories.

Assumptions/Propositions about Nursing

Among the theorists, there are certain assumptions upon which it is clear that they all agree, as well as those upon which many agree or disagree. There are also assumptions upon which they agree, but which they apply differently in terms of nursing care. At times the theorists utilize very similar terms to identify the same phenomena within a given situation. There are also those theorists who agree with each other, and those who disagree a great deal. What is most significant are the assumptions that are supported by most theorists and not contradicted by the others. These provide a strong foundation for practice regardless of the particular theory the nurse is incorporating into her patient care. These, in fact, as interpreted by the author, become her view of nursing's *universal* propositions for practice. (Note Chapter 1.)

Nursing is a discipline distinctly different from but supportive of medicine.

This proposition does not deny that the nurse supports the activities of the physician in terms of assisting in the medical care of patients. What is significant is that nurses require a separate body of nursing and scientific knowledge, integrated in such a way as to facilitate nursing care rather than medical care.

The major focus of nursing is on the human being/individual.

Although this proposition seems self-evident, it should be apparent by now that, starting with Nightingale in 1860 and ending with Watson in 1979, the theorists have constantly attempted to explain the role of thenurse as that of providing care to human beings. Whether the focus is on human needs, human interaction, the environment, or humans within a system, the goal is clear—to assist humans to retain or regain *health*, how ever that is defined.

The greater the understanding of human beings, the more effective the nursing care will be.

Within the theories there is a constant attempt to explain the characteristics of human beings. The greater this understanding, the more successful the nurse will be in achieving nursing goals.

Change as a process relates to all the four major concepts in nursing.

Humans change their behavior and their health state. The *environment* is constantly changing and creating differing forces or stresses with which humans must deal. *Health* is not static but dynamic. During illness, the goal is to change the individual's illness state to a healthier state. *Nursing* activities must be modified as the health state, the environment, and the patient's behaviors change. Because of change, nursing requires continuous observations and new data.

Nursing as a discipline requires content and process.

The content of nursing is projected in the theories as well as within their scientific foundations. The process used to apply this content to the real world of nursing is crucial for quality nursing care. Thus, *content* gives us a frame of reference with which to look at a nursing situation, and *process* provides the way of thinking about, assimilating, or utilizing that content for the achievement of some goal. The old expression that nursing is an art and a science continues to be valid. Now we use the terms *content* for *science* and *process* for *art*.

There are also some propositions about which there is general agreement, with some inconsistencies, among the theories.

Humans are holistic in nature.

Most theorists accept the fact that humans are holistic—integrated wholes in which the parts are inseparable. Others believe that understanding the parts, such as the human biopsychosocial characteristics, aids one in comprehending the whole (whole = the sum of the parts; holism = more than the sum of the parts, but interacting wholes). The literature remains confusing on this point both within the nursing theories and within other writings.

Nursing is basically involved in the care of ill individuals.

Theorists generally agree that the *major* focus of nursing care is the ill individual. Some do emphasize the need for nurses to prevent disease and promote health or assist individuals to achieve a higher degree of human potential. There is also a somewhat limited consideration of the family and the community in many of the theories.

The goal of nursing is to assist individuals to adapt to their illness and the environment.

Many theorists support adaptation as a goal, while others see individual adaptation as a terminal goal and thus a contradiction to the open-systems approach.

The specific concepts also differ among the theorists, but the meanings of the concepts seem quite similar. The word *stress* is frequently used, but its meaning also relates to the concepts *stimuli, force, energy, concern,* and *tension. Need* also relates to *problems, requisites, drives,* or *propensity. Human* is expressed by such terms as *patient, individual, family,* and *nurse.* One theorist might use the word *empathy* to include *sympathy,* while another finds these terms dissimilar and feels that *sympathy* is an inappropriate term to use within the patient-nurse relationship. Many terms—such as *problem solving, phases,* and *scientific decision making*—are used to reflect the nursing process, but the basic approaches remains more similar than dissimilar.

A SELECTED BIBLIOGRAPHY

Abdellah, F.G. "Approaches To Protecting the Rights of Human Subjects." *Nursing Research* (Fall 1967), 316-320.

_____. "Conference On the Nature Of Science In Nursing: The Nature of Nursing Science." *Japanese Journal Of Nursing* (Summer 1970), 248-252.

_____. "Criteria Of Evaluation In Nursing." *Revista Brasileira Enfermagem* (January-February 1973), 17-32.

_____. "Education For Health Services Administration." *American Journal of Public Health* (October 1970), 1890-1891.

_____. "Evolution of Nursing As A Profession: Perspective on Manpower Development." *International Nursing Review* (1972) 219-238.

_____. "Extending the Scope of Nursing Practice." *National League for Nursing Publications* (1972), 1-16.

_____. "Frontiers In Nursing Research." *Nursing Forum* 5:28-38 (1966), 28-38.

_____. "Future Directions: Impact on NSNA 1982 and 2012." *Imprint* (February-March 1983), 66-74.

_____. "Future Directions of the Profession: Impact on NSNA 1982 and 2012. Part II." *Imprint* (April–May 1983), 71–91.

_____. "The Future of Long-term Care." *Bulletin of the New York Academy of Medicine* (March 1978), 261–270.

_____. "Health Care Systems: A Must For Health Care In the 70's." *Journal of Continuing Education in Nursing* (January–February 1971), 10–12.

_____. "Keynote Address: 75th Anniversary of the West Virginia State Nurses' Association." *Weather Vane* (December 1982), 10–13.

_____. "Long-term Care Facility Improvement: A Nationwide Research Effort," *Journal of Long Term Care Administration* (Winter 1976), 5–19.

_____. "Long Term Care—A Top Health Priority." *Journal of Long Term Care Administration* (Spring 1974), 1–3.

_____. "National Library of Medicine Is Official Nursing Archives." *Nursing Research* (January–February 1975), 64.

_____. "A Nationwide Study To Evaluate the Care of Patients In Nursing Homes." *Public Health Reports* (January–February 1977), 30–33.

_____. "The Nature of Nursing Science." *Nursing Research* (September–October 1969), 390–393.

_____. "Nurse Practitioners and Nursing Practice." *American Journal of Public Health* (March 1976), 245–246.

_____. "The Nurse Practitioner 17 Years Later: Present and Emerging Issues." *Inquiry* (Summer 1982), 105–116.

_____. "Nursing and Health Care in the U.S.S.R.." *American Journal of Nursing* (December 1973), 2096–2099.

_____. "The Nursing Archives at the National Library of Medicine." *Nursing Research* (September–October 1975), 0029–6562.

_____. "Nursing Care of the Aged in the United States of America." *Journal of Gerontological Nursing* (November 1981), 657–663.

_____. "1983–2008: Nursing Practice." *Arizona Nurse* (March–April 1983), 6–7.

_____. "Nursing Problems in Long-term Care and Nursing Education." *Kango* (July 1977), 139–146.

_____. "Nursing Research in the Health Services." *Nursing Research Report* (December 1969), 2.

_____. "Nursing's Role in Future Health Care." *Association of Operating Room Nurses* (August 1976), 236–240.

_____. "An Overview of Nurse-scientist Programs in the Country." *National League for Nursing Publications* (1968), 11-24.

_____. "Overview of Nursing Research 1955-1968. 1." *Nursing Research* (January-February 1970), 6-17.

_____. "Overview of Nursing Research 1955-1968. 3." *Nursing Research* (May-June 1970), 239-252.

_____. "The Physician-Nurse Team Approach to Coronary Care." *Nursing Clinics of North America* (September 1972), 423-430.

_____. "Preparing For the Health Care Issues of the 1980s." *National League for Nursing Publications* (1979), 1-11.

_____. "Problems, Issues, Challenges of Nursing Research." *Canada Nurse* (May 1971), 44-6.

_____. "Research on Career Development in the Health Professions: Nursing." *Occupational Health Nursing* (May 1973), 12-16.

_____. "School Nurse Practitioner: An Expanded Role For Nurses." *Journal of American College Health* (June 1973), 423-432.

_____. "Search or Research? An Experiment To Stimulate Research." *Nursing Outlook* (October 1965), 65-67.

_____. "Training and Development of the Health Care Team." *Association of Operating Room Nurses* (May 1970). 86-91.

_____. "U.S. Public Health Service's Contribution to Nursing Research: Past, Present, Future." *Nursing Research* (July-August 1977), 0029-6562.

Abdellah, F.G., F.T. Billings, R.O. Egeberg, A.E. Hess, J.E. Muller, and D. Petit. "The Soviet Health System: Aspects of Relevance For Medicine in the United States." *New England Journal of Medicine* (March 1972), 693-702.

Abdellah, F.G., and R.K. Chow. "The Long-term Care Facility Improvement Campaign: The PACE Project." *Association of Rehabilitation Nurses* (November-December 1976), 3-4.

Abdellah, F.G., R.K. Chow, and H.V. Foerst. "PACEL: An Approach to Improving the Care of the Elderly." *American Journal of Nursing* (June 1979), 1109-1110.

Abdellah, F.G., and M.E. Levine. "The Aims of Nursing Research." *Comprehensive Nursing Quarterly* (Summer 1968), 12-31.

_____. "Better Patient Care Through Nursing Research (1)." *Kango Tenbo* (August 1982), 714-719).

_____. "Better Patient Care Through Nursing Research: Progress In the Study Of Patient Classification (3)." *Kango Tenbo* (October 1982), 916-921.

_____. "Future Directions of Research In Nursing." *American Journal of Nursing* (January 1966), 112-116.

_____. "Progress In the Studies of Patient Classification." *Kango Tenbo* (September 1982), 819-823.

Abdellah, F.G., and J.D. Matarazzo. "Doctoral Education For Nurses in the United States." *Nursing Research* (September-October 1971), 404-414.

Carozza, V., J. Congdon, and J. Watson. "An Experimental Educationally Sponsored Pilot Internship Program." *Journal of Nursing Education* (November 1978), 14-20.

Chinn, P., and M. Jacobs. *Theory and Nursing: A Systematic Approach.* St. Louis, Mo.: The C.V. Mosby Company, 1983.

Cupoli, A., B. Corvine, M. Horwitz, E. Kudzma, M.J. Midura, S. Mott, K.S. Ramos, and J. Watson. "Postpartum Teaching Regarding Infant Care, Behavior, and Characteristics: A Study." *Bulletin of the American College Nurse Midwife* (November 1971), 112-121.

Daubenmire, M.J., and I.M. King. "Nursing Process Models: A Systems Approach." *Nursing Outlook* (August 1973), 512-517.

Deloughery, G.W., K.M. Gebbie, and B.M. Neuman. "Change In Problem-solving Ability Among Nurses Receiving Mental Health Consultation." *Communicating Nursing Research* (September 1970), 41-53.

_____. "Levels of Utilization: Nursing Specialists In Community Mental Health." *Journal of Psychiatric Nursing* (January-February 1970), 37-39.

_____. "Teaching Organizational Concepts To Nurses In Community Mental Health." *Journal of Nursing Education* (January 1974), 8-14.

Dickoff, J., P. James, and E. Wiedenbach. "Theory in a Practice Discipline: Practice Oriented Discipline." Part 1. *Nursing Research* (September-October 1968), 415-435.

_____. "Theory in a Practice Discipline: Practice Oriented Research." Part 2. *Nursing Research* (November-December 1968), 545-554.

Fulp, E.M., and M.E. Rogers. "N.C. Nurses Visit China Health Services for a Billion People." *Tar Hael Nurse* (November-December 1982), 5, 8.

Gabriel, F.D., M.E. Levine, and F. Rosner. "Leukemoid Reactions With Extreme Thrombocytosis." *New York Journal of Medicine* (June 1970), 1314-1318.

Hall, L.E. "Another View of Nursing Care and Quality." *Maryland Nurse* (Spring 1968), 2-12.

_____. "The Loeb Center For Nursing and Rehabilitation, Montefiore Hospital and Medical Center, Bronx, New York." *International Journal of Nursing Studies* (July 1969), 81-97.

Heller, M.P., and Imogene M. King. "Team Teaching: Values and Advantages." *Nursing Outlook* (October 1965), 50-51.

Henderson, P.A., and V. Henderson. "Teamwork In Maternity and Infant Care Projects." *Obstetrics and Gynecology* (March 1972), 401-406.

Henderson, V. "Awareness of Library Resources: A Characteristic of Professional Workers; An Essential in Research and Continuing Education." *American Nurses' Association Publications* (1977), 1-15.

_____. "Basic Principles of Nursing Care." *Korean Nurse* (April 1970), 29-33.

_____. "Basic Principles of Nursing Care." *Korean Nurse* (February 1970), 33-37.

_____. "Basic Principles of Nursing Care. 2." *Korean Nurse* (August 1969), 45-49.

_____. "Basic Principles of Nursing Care. 3." *Korean Nurse* (October 1969), 51-56.

_____. "Basic Principles of Nursing Care. 4." *Korean Nurse* (December 1969), 69-73.

_____. "The Concept of Nursing." *Journal of Advanced Nursing* (March 1978), 113-130.

_____. "Defining Nursing—Identifying 'Nursing Theory,' 'Nursing Science,' and 'The Nursing Process'—An Interpretation," *Kango* (January 1983), 10-31.

_____. "The Essence of Nursing in an Age of Technology (Interview)." *Professioni Infermierstiche* (October-December 1980), 170-173.

_____. "Excellence in Nursing." *American Journal of Nursing* (October 1969), 2133-2137.

_____. "Excellence in Nursing." *Comprehensive Nursing Quarterly* (Spring 1970), 21-33.

_____. "Health Is Everybody's Business." *Canadian Nurse* (March 1971), 31-34.

_____. "Health Personnel As Assistants To Patients—Or People." *Virginia Nurse Quarterly* (Winter 1971), 9.

_____. "Implications For Nursing In the Library Activities of the Regional Medical Programs." *Bulletin of the Medical Library Association* (January 1971), 53-64.

_____. "An Interview With Miss Virginia Henderson. Nurses' Actions: Definition by Henderson and That of Nightingale." *Kango* (December 1982), 30-48.

_____. "Interview With Virginia Henderson." *Revista de Enfermagem* (December 1981, January 1982), 38-40.

_____. "Is The Role of the Nurse Changing?" *Weather Vane* (October 1968), 12-13.

_____. "Library Resources In Nursing: Their Development and Use." Part 1. *International Nursing Review* (April 1968), 164-182.

_____. "Library Resources In Nursing—Their Development and Use." Part 2. *International Nursing Review* (July 1968), 236-47.

_____. "Library Resources In Nursing—Their Development and Use." Part 3. *International Nursing Review* (October 1968), 348-358.

_____. "The Nursing Process—Is the Title Right?" *Journal of Advanced Nursing* (March 1982), 103-109.

_____. "Nursing Research—Notes On Its Development and Current Status—A Special Speech Delivered by Virginia Henderson." *Kango* (December 1982), 4-29.

_____. "Nursing—Yesterday and Tomorrow." *Nursing Times* (May 22, 1980), 905-7.

_____. "On Nursing Care Plans and Their History." *Nursing Outlook* (June 1973), 378-379.

_____. "Preserving the Essence of Nursing in a Technological Age." *Nursing Times* (November 29, 1979), 2056-2058.

_____. "Preserving the Essence of Nursing in a Technological Age." *Kango Kyoiku* (May 1980), 293-301.

_____. "Professional Writing." *Nursing Mirror* (May 1978), 15-18.

_____. "70 Plus and Going Strong: Virginia Henderson, A Nurse For All Ages." *Geriatric Nursing* (January-February 1983), 58-59.

_____. "Some Commitments For Nurses Today." *Alumnae Magazine* (Spring 1968), 5-15.

_____. "We've 'Come A Long Way,' But What of the Direction?" *Nursing Research* (May-June 1977), 163-164.

_____. "Yesterday and Tomorrow of Nursing." *Revista Enfermagem* (September 1982), 6-8.

Henderson, Virginia, and S. Watt. "Epidermolysis Bullosa." *Nursing Times* (June 29-July 5, 1983), 43-46.

Holloway, E., and I.M. King. "What's Going On Here?" *Nursing Research* (September-October 1983), 319-320.

Inada, Y., H. Peplau, and N. Tsuzki. "Interview With Dr. Peplau: Future of Nursing." *Japanese Journal of Nursing* (October 1975), 1046-1050.

Johnson, D. "Abuse of the Elderly." *Nurse Practitioner* (January-February 1981), 29-34.

_____. "Cardiovascular Care in the First Person." *ANA Clinical Session* (1972), 127-134.

_____. "Competence in Practice: Technical and Professional." *Nursing Outlook* (October 1966), 30-33.

_____. "Development of Theory: A Requisite For Nursing As a Primary Health Profession." *Nursing Research* (September-October 1974), 0029-6562.

_____. "A High Privilege To Be Real." *Christian Nurse* (June 1968), 8-13.

_____. "The Nature of a Science of Nursing." *Comprehensive Nursing Quarterly* (January 1967), 56-66.

_____. "State of the Art of Theory Development In Nursing." *National League for Nursing Publications* (1978), 1-10.

_____. "Symposium On Theory Development In Nursing. Theory In Nursing: Borrowed and Unique." *Nursing Research* (May-June 1968), 206-209.

_____. "Today's Action Will Determine Tomorrow's Nursing." *Nursing Outlook* (September 1965), 38-41.

Johnson, D., H.C. Moidel, and J.A. Wilcox. "The Clinical Specialist As A Practitioner." *American Journal of Nursing* (November 1967), 2298-2303.

King, I.M. "A Conceptual Frame of Reference for Nursing." *Nursing Research* (January-February 1968), 27-31.

_____. "How Does the Conceptual Framework Provide Structure For the Curriculum?" *National League for Nursing Publications* (1978), 23-34.

_____. "Planning For Change." *Ohio Nurses Review* (August 1970), 4-7.

_____. "Toward the Future In Nursing Research." *Communicating Nursing Research* (1968), 158-166.

_____. "U.S.A.: Loyola University of Chicago School of Nursing." *Journal of Advanced Nursing* (July 1978), 390.

_____. "The 'Why' of Theory Development." *National League for Nursing Publications* (1978), 11-16.

King, I.M., and M. Sugimori. "A Special Interview: Dr. Imogene M. King." *Kango Kyoiku* (October 1977), 597-602.

King, I.M., and B. Tarsitano. "The Effect of Structured and Unstructured Pre-operative Teaching: A Replication." *Nursing Research* (November–December 1982), 324-329.

Lambertsen, E., M.E. Rogers, Sr. M. Margaret, and C.E. O'Neil. "Action-reaction; Four NYSNA Members React to the ANA Position Paper on Education." *New York State Nurse* (May 1966), 6-8.

Levine, E.B., and M.E. Levine. "Hippocrates, Father of Nursing, Too?" *American Journal of Nursing* (December 1965), 86-88.

Levine, M.E. "Adaptation and Assessment: A Rationale For Nursing Intervention." *American Journal of Nursing* (November 1966), 2450-2453.

_____. "Benoni." *American Journal of Nursing* (March 1972), 466-468.

_____. "Bioethics of Cancer Nursing." *Association of Rehabilitation Nurses* (March–April 1982), 27-31.

_____. "Breaking Through the Medications Mystique." *American Journal of Nursing* (April 1970), 799-803.

_____. "Cancer Chemotherapy—A Nursing Model." *Nursing Clinics Of North America* (June 1978), 271-280.

_____. "Does Continuing Education Improve Nursing Practice?" *Hospitals* (November 1978), 138-140.

_____. "The Ethics of Computer Technology In Health Care." *Nursing Forum* (1980), 193-198.

_____. "Florence Nightingale: The Legend That Lives." *Comprehensive Nursing Quarterly* (Fall 1971), 38-46.

_____. "The Four Conservation Principles of Nursing." *Nursing Forum* (1967), 45-59.

_____. "Holistic Nursing." *Nursing Clinics of North America* (June 1971), 253-264.

_____. "The Intransigent Patient." *American Journal of Nursing* (October 1970), 2106-2111.

_____. "Introduction of Exchange Transfusion." *New England Journal of Medicine* (November 1971), 1152.

_____. "Knock Before Entering Personal Space Bubbles. 1." *Chart* (February 1968), 58-62.

_____. "Knock Before Entering Personal Space Bubbles. II." *Chart* (March 1968), 82-84.

_____. "Knowledge Base Required By General and Specialized Nursing Practice." *American Nurses' Association Publications* (1977), 57-69.

_____. "Nursing Ethics and the Ethical Nurse." *American Journal of Nursing* (May 1977), 845-849.

_____. "On Creativity In Nursing." *Image* (1973), 15-19.

_____. "Patients and Practice." *Registered Nurses' Association of Ontario News* (June-July 1973), 19-21.

_____. "Psychotherapy of Borderline Patients." *American Journal of Psychiatry* (November 1968), 704-705.

_____. "The Pursuit of Wholeness." *American Journal of Nursing* (January 1969), 93-98.

_____. "Small Hospital—Big Nursing." *Chart* (October 1969), 265-269.

_____. "Small Hospital—Big Nursing." Part 2. *Chart* (November 1969), 310-315.

_____. "This I Believe . . . About Patient-centered Care." *Nursing Outlook* (July 1967), 53-55.

_____. "Time Has Come To Speak of . . . Health Care." *Association of Operating Room Nurses* (June 1971), 37-43.

Loetterle, B.C., M. Rogers, T. Valdner, C. Mason, I. Christian, and W. Anderson. "Cerebellar Stimulation: Pacing the Brain." *American Journal of Nursing* (June 1975), 958-960.

McNeill, R.S., and J.M. Watson. "Oxygen Therapy in the Home" *British Medical Journal* (February 1966), 331-333.

Neuman, B., and M. Wyatt. "Prospects For Change: Some Evaluative Reflections From One Articulated Baccalaureate Program." *Journal of Nursing Education* (January 1981), 40-46.

Neuman, B.M., and R.J. Young. "A Model For Teaching Total Person Approach To Patient Problems." *Nursing Research* (May-June 1972), 264-269.

Nightingale, F. "Introductory Notes On Lying-in Institutions By Florence Nightingale." *Sogo Kango* (1983), 59-73.

_____. "Introductory Notes On Lying-in Institutions Part 2." *Sogo Kango* (May 15, 1983), 113-130.

_____. "Letter To the Nurses of the Nightingale Fund School." *Caridad Ciencia y Arte* (January-March 1971), 3-4.

_____. "Looking Back: Taken From 'Notes On Hospitals' By Florence Nightingale, 1863." *Lamp* (September 1979), 39-43.

_____. "Notes On Hospitals. 2. 1: Hygienic Conditions of the Hospital." *Comprehensive Nursing Quarterly* (Summer 1970), 88-97.

_____. "Notes On Hospitals. 5." *Comprehensive Nursing Quarterly* (Spring 1971), 87-98.

_____. "Notes On Hospitals. 6. Three Basic Rules On Hospital Architecture." *Comprehensive Nursing Quarterly* (Summer 1971), 72-81.

_____. "Notes On Hospitals. 7." *Comprehensive Nursing Quarterly* (Fall 1971), 86-98.

_____. "Notes On Hospitals. 9. (IV). Improved Hospital Plans: V. A Hospital For Convalescence." *Comprehensive Nursing Quarterly* (Summer 1972), 89-99.

_____. "Notes On Hospitals. (11). VI. Children's Hospitals. VII. Military Hospitals In India." *Comprehensive Nursing Quarterly* (Spring 1973), 82-93.

_____. "Notes On Nursing: What It Is and What It Is Not. 1." *Comprehensive Nursing Quarterly* (Spring 1974), 92-98.

_____. "Notes On Nursing: What It Is and What It Is Not. 2." *Comprehensive Nursing Quarterly* (Summer 1974), 85-99.

_____. "Notes On Nursing. V. Convalescent Hospitals. VI. Pediatric Hospitals." *Comprehensive Nursing Quarterly* (Winter 1972), 86-97.

Orem, D.E. "From American Nursing Research." *Sykepleien* (April 1970), 244-245.

_____. "Levels of Nursing Education and Practice." *Alumnae Magazine* (March 1969), 2-6.

Peplau, H.E. "The A.N.A. and Nursing Education." *Utah Nurse* (Fall 1969), 6.

_____. "A.N.A. and the Professional Nurse." *National League for Nursing Publications* (1974), 26-28.

_____. "ANA—Who Needs It?" *Nursing News* (December 1970), 5-8.

_____. "ANA—Who Needs It? Part 2." *Nursing News* (January 1971), 12-14.

_____. "Changed Patterns of Practice." *Washington State Journal of Nursing* (November-December 1970), 4-6.

_____. "The Changing View of Nursing." *International Nursing Review* (March-April 1977), 43-45.

_____. "Creativity and Commitment In Nursing." *Image* (1974), 13-15.

_____. "Dilemmas of Organizing Nurses." *Image* (1971), 4-8.

_____. "The Independence of Nursing." *Imprint* (May 1972), 11.

_____. "An Interpretation of the ANA Position." *New Jersey State Nurses' Association Newsletter* (March–April 1966), 6–10.

_____. "In Support of Nursing Research." *Journal of the New York State Nurses Association* (Spring 1971), 5.

_____. "Is Health Care a Right? Affirmative Response." *Image* (1974), 4–10.

_____. "Keynote Address at 68th Annual Convention of NJSNA." *NJSNA Newsletter* (November–December 1970), 3–10.

_____. "Meeting the Challenge." *Miss R.N.* (July 1973), 1–6.

_____. "Mid-Life Crises." *American Journal of Nursing* (October 1975), 1761–1765.

_____. "The Now Nurse in Nursing: Some Problems of Diversity." *Oklahoma Nurse* (November 1971), 46.

_____. "The Nurse in the Community Mental Health Program." *Nursing Outlook* (November 1965), 68–70.

_____. "Nurse-Doctor Relationships." *Nursing Forum* (1966), 5:60–75 #1 (1966).

_____. "Nurses: Collaborate or Isolate." *Pennsylvania Nurse* (January 1974), 2–5.

_____. "The Nurse's Role in Health Care Delivery Systems." *Pelican News* (Spring 1972), 12–14.

_____. "Nursing: The Heart of Health Care." *Bulletin of the Massachusetts Nurses Association* (Summer 1971), 3–5.

_____. "Nursing's Two Routes to Doctoral Degrees." *Nursing Forum* (1966), 57–67.

_____. "Professional Closeness—As a Special Kind of Involvement with a Patient, Client, or Family Group." *Nursing Forum* (1969), 342–360.

_____. "Psychotherapeutic Strategies." *Perspectives in Psychiatric Care* (November–December, 1968), 264–270.

_____. "The Psychiatric Nurse—Accountable? To Whom? For What?" *Perspectives in Psychiatric Care* (May–June 1980), 128–134.

_____. "Psychiatric Nursing: Role of Nurses and Psychiatric Nurses." *International Nursing Review* (March–April 1978), 41–47.

_____. "Theory: The Professional Dimension." *Proceedings of the Nursing Theory Conference* (March 1969), 33–46.

_____. "Responsibility, Authority, Evaluation and Accountability of Nursing in Patient Care." *Michigan Nurse* (July 1971), 5–7.

_____. "The Road Ahead." *Maine Nurse* (December 1970), 3–8.

_____. "Some Reflections on Earlier Days in Psychiatric Nursing." *Journal of Psychosocial Nursing and Mental Health Services* (August 1982), 17–24.

_____. "Talking With Patients." *Comprehensive Nurse Quarterly* (Autumn 1974), 30–39.

_____. "A Task Ahead." *American Journal of Nursing* (September 1971), 1800.

_____. "Time of Decision." *Nevada Nurses Association Quarterly Newsletter* (Summer 1971), 1–3.

_____. "Trends in Nursing and Nursing Education." *New Jersey Student Nursing Association Newsletter* (May–June 1966), 17–27.

_____. "What it Means to be a Professional Nurse in Today's Society." *Kansas Nurse* (November 1971), 1–3.

_____. "What it Means to be a Professional Nurse Today." *Alabama Nurse* (December 1970), 8–17.

_____. "Where Do We Go From Here?" *Pelican News* (Winter 1971), 14–16.

Rogers, M.E. "Collegiate Education in Nursing." *Nursing Science* (October 1965), 362–365.

_____. "Contemporary American Leaders in Nursing; An Oral History. 3. Martha E. Rogers Interviewed." *Kango Tenbo* (December 1979), 1126–1138.

_____. "Doctoral Education in Nursing." *Nursing Forum* (2, 1966), 5:75–82.

_____. "Euphemisms in Nursing's Future." *Image* (2, 1975), 7:3–9.

_____. "Higher Education in Nursing." *Nursing Science* (December 1965), 443–445.

_____. "Legislative and Licensing Problems in Health Care." *Nursing Administration Quarterly* (Spring 1978), 71–78.

_____. "New Designs—Experiments In Action." *National League for Nursing Conference of the Council of Member Agencies of the Department of Bacculaureate and Higher Degree Program Papers* (1966), 23–26.

_____. "Nursing Concepts." *Korean Nurse* (August 1975), 36–37.

_____. "Nursing Education for Professional Practice." *Catholic Nurse* (September 1969), 28–37.

_____. "Nursing's Expanding Role and Other Euphemisms." *Journal of the New York State Nurses Association* (December 1972), 5–10.

_____. "Nursing is Coming of Age . . . Through the Practitioner Movement (Con)." *American Journal of Nursing* (October 1975), 1834–1843.

_____. "Nursing Research: Relevant to Practice?" *Nursing Research Conference* (March 1969), 352–359.

_____. "Nursing: To Be or Not to Be?" *Nursing Outlook* (January 1972), 42–46.

_____. "Preparation of the Baccalaureate Degree Graduate." *National Journal Student Nurses Association* (November-December 1969), 32–37.

_____. "Quality Nursing—Cliche or Challenge?" *Maine Nurse* (Winter 1966), 2–4.

_____. "Reactions to the Two Foregoing Presentations." *National League for Nursing Publications* (1972), 62–65. No. 15-1456.

_____. "Ribonucleoprotein Particles in the Amphibian Oocyte Nucleus: Possible Intermediates in Ribosome Synthesis." *Journal of Cell Biology* (March 1968), 421–432.

_____. "Yesterday a Nurse, Tomorrow a Manager; What Now?" *Journal of the New York State Nurses Association* (Spring 1970), 15–21.

Rogers, M.E., U.E. Loening, and R.S. Frasser. "Ribosomal RNA Precursors in Plants." *Journal of Molecular Biology* (May 1970), 681–692.

Roy, C. "Adaptation: A Basis for Nursing Practice." *Nursing Outlook* (April 1971), 254–257.

_____. "Adaptation: A Conceptual Framework for Nursing." *Nursing Outlook* (March 1970), 42–45.

_____. "A Diagnostic Classification System for Nursing." *Nursing Outlook* (February 1975), 90–94.

_____. "The Future of Nursing." *National League for Nursing Publication* (1979), 3–19.

_____. "Home Hemodialysis and the Older Patient." *Journal of the American Association of Nephrologic Nurses Technician* (1980), 317–324.

_____. "The Impact of Nursing Diagnosis." *Journal of the Association of Operating Room Nurses* (May 1975), 1023–1030.

_____. "Relating Nursing Theory to Education: A New Era." *Nurse Education* (March–April 1979), 16–21.

_____. "Role Cues for the Mother of the Hospitalized Child." *American Nursing Association* (1968), 199–206.

_____. "The Roy Adaptation Model: Comment." *Nursing Outlook* (November 1976), 690-691.

Roy, C., and M. Obloy. "The Practitioner Movement: Toward a Science of Nursing." *American Journal of Nursing* (October 1978), 1698-1702.

Roy, C., and M. Shurr. "The Home Hemodialysis Assistant: Outpatient Groups." *Nephrologic Nurse* (September 1981), 39-44.

Sanford, R., and M. Rogers. "The SAIN Alternative: An Interview with Martha Rogers." *Journal of Nursing Care* (July 1978), 20-23.

Tannenbaum, R.P., C.A. Sohn, R. Cantwell, M. Rogers, and R. Hollis. "Pain: Angina Pectoris: How to Recognize It; How to Manage It." *Nursing* (September 1981), 44-51.

Wang, R.Y., and J. Watson. "The Professional Nurse: Roles, Competencies and Characteristics." *Supervisory Nurse* (June 1977), 69-71.

Watson, J. "Conceptual Systems of Undergraduate Nursing Students as Compared with University Students at Large and Practicing Nurses." *Nursing Research* (May-June 1978), 151-155.

_____. "Conceptual System, Students, Practitioners." *Western Journal of Nursing Research* (Spring 1981), 172-198.

_____. "Death Revisited." *Perspective in Psychiatric Care* (United States) (April-June 1974), 73.

_____. "Ethical Issues in Nursing and Health Sciences: Emerging Issues and Conflicts for Nurses." *Australian Nurses Journal* (December-January 1983), 94-96.

_____. "The Evolution of Nursing Education in the United States: 100 Years of a Profession for Women." *Journal of Nursing Education* (September 1977), 31-38.

_____. "Existentialism: Its Relevance for Practice and Education." *Supervisory Nurse* (February 1975), 21, 23-27.

_____. "How Does a Nurse Interested in Research Identify a Researchable Question?" *Nursing Research* (November-December 1976), 439.

_____. "How to Select Clinical Agencies for Clinical Experiences in Baccalaureate Nursing Education." *Journal of Nursing Education* (February 1979), 29-35.

_____. "The Lost Art of Nursing." *Nursing Forum* (1981), 244-249.

_____. "Nursing's Scientific Quest." *Nursing Outlook* (July 1981), 413-416.

_____. "Patient Evaluation of a Primary Nursing Project." *Australian Journal of Nursing* (November 1978), 30-33.

_____. "President's Page. Nurses and Doctors." *Australian Family Physician* (April 1977), 4.

_____. "Primary Nursing—Nursing Care Can be Patient Centered." *Australian Journal of Nursing* (August 1977), 35-39.

_____. "Professional Identity Crisis: Is Nursing Finally Growing Up?" *American Journal of Nursing* (August 1981), 488-490.

_____. "Research and Literature on Children's Responses to Injections: Some General Nursing Implications." *Pediatric Nurse* (January-February 1975), 7-8.

_____. "Role Conflict in Nursing." *Supervisory Nurse* (July 1977), 40-41.

_____. "Traditional v. Tertiary: Ideological Shifts in Nursing Education." *Australian Nurses Journal* (August 1982), 44-46.

_____. "Treatment and Nursing of the Severely Burned Patient." *Nursing Mirror* (January 1970), 13-15.

Watson, J., C. Burckhardt, L. Brown, D. Bloch, and N. Hester. "A Model of Caring: An Alternative Health Care Model for Nursing Practice and Research." *American Nursing Association Publication* (1979), 32-44.

Wiedenbach, E. "Comment on 'Beliefs and Values: Bases for Curriculum Design'." *Nursing Research* (September-October 1970), 427.

_____. "Family Nurse Practitioner for Maternal and Child Care." *Nursing Outlook* (December 1965), 50-52.

_____. "Genetics and the Nurse." *Bulletin of the American College Nurse Midwife* (May 1968), 8-13.

_____. "The Nurse's Role in Family Planning: A Conceptual Basis for Practice." *Nursing Clinics of North America* (June 1968), 355-365.

_____. "Nurses' Wisdom in Nursing Theory." *American Journal of Nursing* (May 1970), 1057-1062.

INDEX

Introduction to Clinical Nursing (Levine), 11 *tab.*

J

Johnson, Dorothy E., theory of, 120-26
application to nursing process, 123, 124-25 *tab.*
basic components, 118 *tab.*
characteristics, 162 *tab.*
compared to King, 135; to Neuman, 145; to Rogers, 128; to Roy, 151
concepts, 122-23
description, 120-21
evaluation, 123-26
focus, 11 *tab.*, 207
major theme, 4 *tab.*, 5, 113 *tab.*
models, 121-22
nursing role and function, 6 *tab.*
Jones, P., 38
Jung, Carl, 51

K

King, Imogene, theory of, 134-42, 166
application to nursing process, 138-41
basic components, 118 *tab.*
characteristics, 163 *tab.*, 164
compared to Abdellah, 82; to Neuman, 147
description, 134-36
evaluation, 141-42
focus, 13 *tab.*, 36 *tab.*
major theme, 4 *tab.*, 5, 113 *tab.*, 211

model, 136-38
nursing role and function, 6 *tab.*
Kinlein, M. Lucille, theory of, 105-8
application to nursing process, 107
description, 105-6
evaluation, 108
focus, 15 *tab.*, 64 *tab.*
major theme, 4 *tab.*, 50 *tab.*
models, 106-7
and need concept, 51 *tab.*, 63, 65, 108, 109, 110
nursing role and function, 6 *tab.*
Knowledge, concept, 83, 88. *See also* Nursing knowledge

L

Learning theory, 166
Leone, Lucille Petry, 179
Levine, E., 78
Levine, Myra Estrin, theory of, 181-89
application to nursing process, 16, 185-88
description, 181-82
evaluation, 188-89
focus, 11 *tab.*, 203 *tab.*
major theme, 4 *tab.*, 167 *tab.*, 204, 211
model, 182-85
nursing role and function, 6 *tab.*
Light, concept, 41, 44, 47, 48
Limitations, concept, 73
Linear-directional models, 24, 25, 26, 32, 76
Living organisms, concept, 116
Living systems, concept, 151-52